Diagnosis and Treatment of Traumatic Injuries to the Pediatric Craniofacial Skeleton

Diagnosis and Treatment of Traumatic Injuries to the Pediatric Craniofacial Skeleton

Charles E. Moore

PLURAL PUBLISHING
INC.
5521 Ruffin Road
San Diego, CA 92123

e-mail: info@pluralpublishing.com
Web site: http://www.pluralpublishing.com

49 Bath Street
Abingdon, Oxfordshire OX14 1EA
United Kingdom

Typeset in 10.5/13 Adobe Garamond Pro by So Cal Graphics
Printed in Hong Kong by Paramount

ISBN-13: **978-1-59756-140-2**
ISBN-10: **1-59756-140-1**

Library of Congress Cataloging-in-Publication Data

Diagnosis and treatment of traumatic injuries to the pediatric craniofacial skeleton /
[edited by] Charles E. Moore.
p. ; cm.
ISBN-13: 978-1-59756-140-2 (hardcover)
ISBN-10: 1-59756-140-1 (hardcover)
1. Face—Wounds and injuries—Surgery. 2. Facial bones—Wounds and injuries—Surgery. 3. Children—Wounds and injuries—Surgery. 4. Fractures in children—Surgery. I. Moore, Charles E. (Charles Earl), 1965-
[DNLM: 1. Facial Injuries—diagnosis. 2. Facial Injuries—therapy. 3. Child. 4. Infant. 5. Reconstructive Surgical Procedures. 6. Skull Fractures—diagnosis. 7. Skull Fractures—therapy. WE 706 D536 2007]
RD523.D47 2007
617.5'2059—dc22

2007018613

Diagnosis and Treatment of Traumatic Injuries to the Pediatric Craniofacial Skeleton

Table of Contents

Preface

The goal of the physician in training and practicing specialist is to pursue the best pathway that leads to preservation of form and function which will ultimately lead to the restoration of health. *Diagnosis and Treatment of Traumatic Injuries to the Pediatric Craniofacial Skeleton* is designed to incite thoughtful consideration of the concepts necessary to accomplish this goal.

A variety of health care professionals may be presented with pediatric patients that have experienced traumatic craniofacial injuries. Therefore, a primary focus of this text is to represent the perspectives of several different specialties. As new diagnostic procedures and methods of treatment continue to evolve, close evaluation of advances such as the technique of approach, the use of materials to accomplish reconstruction, and consideration of imaging techniques are critical to accomplishing the best reconstructive goals. This text exposes the reader to a discussion of issues pertinent to pediatric facial trauma from the viewpoint of an oral surgeon, neurosurgeon, dentist, ophthalmologist, otolaryngologist, radiologist, plastic surgeon, and craniomaxillofacial surgeon. Close cooperation among all those working in the various related disciplines and specialties for the craniomaxillofacial area is essential to ensure optimal results for patients.

Given that there are many ways to achieve the desired results in medicine and surgery, continuous exposure to new and innovative concepts is essential to provide the best care to the pediatric patient. *Diagnosis and Treatment of Traumatic Injuries to the Pediatric Craniofacial Skeleton* endeavors to compile the current concepts and thereby create a canvas through descriptions and illustrations pertaining to examination, diagnosis, and treatment that provides guidelines for the diagnosis and treatment of the pediatric patient.

About the Editor

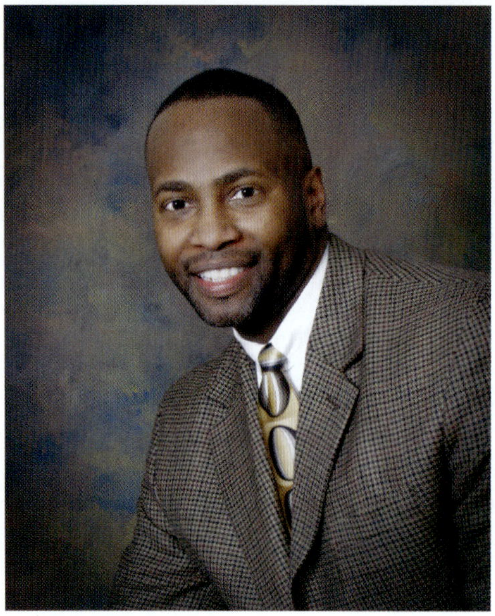

Dr. Charles E. Moore is a graduate of Harvard Medical School. He completed a general surgery internship, otolaryngology residency, and fellowship at the University of Michigan. His fellowship training was in Craniomaxillofacial-Cranial Base and Facial Plastic and Reconstructive Surgery. He is board certified and currently serves on the faculty of the Emory University Medical Center in Atlanta, Georgia. He is also the Chief of Service in the Department of Otolaryngology at Grady Memorial Hospital in Atlanta, Georgia.

Contributors

Diagnosis and Treatment of Traumatic Injuries to the Pediatric Craniofacial Skeleton

Contributors

Russell Ashinoff, MD
Emory University Hospital
Grady Health System
Atlanta, Ga
Chapter 3

C. Robert Bernardino, MD, FACS
Director, Ophthalmic Plastic and Orbital Surgery
Yale Eye Center
New Haven, Conn
Chapter 4

Amanda Corey, MD
Department of Radiology
Emory University
Atlanta, GA
Chapters 8 & 9

Frederick Durden, MD
Emory University Hospital
Grady Health System
Atlanta, Ga
Chapter 8

Michael P. Healey, DDS
Academy of General Dentistry
Dunwoody, Ga
Chapter 6

Albert Losken, MD
Emory University Hospital
Emory Crawford Long Hospital
Atlanta VA Medical Center
Grady Memorial Hospital
Children's Healthcare of Atlanta at Egleston
The Emory Clinic
Atlanta, Ga
Chapter 3

Charles E. Moore, MD
Chief of Service, Otolaryngology Clinic, Grady Health System
Otolaryngology Department, Emory Healthcare
Children's Healthcare of Atlanta at Egleston
Children's Healthcare of Atlanta at Hughes Spaulding
Atlanta, Ga
Chapter 1

Carrie Muh, MD
Emory University School of Medicine
Deptartment of Neurosurgery
Atlanta, Ga
Chapter 7

Steven Roser, MD
Emory University Hospital
Emory Crawford Long Hospital
Atlanta VA Medical Center
Grady Memorial Hospital
Children's Healthcare of Atlanta at Egleston
The Emory Clinic
Atlanta, Ga
Chapter 5

Martin B. Steed, DDS
Emory University Hospital
Emory Crawford Long Hospital
Atlanta VA Medical Center
Grady Memorial Hospital
Children's Healthcare of Atlanta at Egleston
The Emory Clinic
Atlanta, Ga
Chapter 2

David Wrubel, MD
Emory University
Children's Healthcare of Atlanta at Egleston
Atlanta, Ga
Chapter 7

Jodi D. Zuckerman, MD
Emory University
Grady Health System
Atlanta, Ga
Chapter 1

This book is dedicated to my teachers, colleagues, and students who are committed to excellence in medicine. Special gratitude goes to my family and friends for their continued support and encouragement.

1

Airway Issues in Pediatric Trauma

Jodi D. Zuckerman
Charles E. Moore

Trauma patients can present with numerous devastating and distracting injuries. It is of utmost importance to always focus on the initial assessment of the trauma patient prior to providing attention to associated traumatic fractures and bleeding. It is essential in pediatric patients to consider the airway prior to beginning any treatment in the initial assessment. Patients may even present with a coexisting airway disorder in the face of other traumatic injuries.

Evaluation of any trauma patient should begin with the essential primary survey. The primary survey should consist of:

A. Airway maintenance with cervical spine protection

B. Breathing and ventilation

C. Circulation and hemorrhage control

D. Disability: Neurologic status

E. Exposure/Environmental control[1]

This chapter focuses on the initial differential for airway obstruction and effective methods to airway maintenance in the trauma patient. It is important to be prepared initially to evaluate the airway in a systematic fashion. The protocol in Figure 1–1 has been developed to assist primary responders in preparation for airway evaluations. By following the steps of the protocol and obtaining the information vital in the historical portion during the initial assessment, the appropriate consultant can be contacted for assistance with the airway. In the face of mandibular fractures, it is important to determine if assistance will be needed for nasotracheal intubation. In midface fractures and trauma to the larynx, it should be determined if oral intubation is possible or if a surgical airway must be attempted to secure the airway. In the setting of a midface fracture, nasotracheal intubation may be contraindicated depending on the location of the fracture(s).

The graphic in Figure 1–2 demonstrates the anatomic location and differential diagnosis of airway obstruction. Nasal fractures, mandibular fractures, maxillary fractures, laryngeal fractures, and penetrating neck trauma can all contribute to respiratory obstruction. The differential diagnosis for airway obstruction in children should be considered a critical aspect of the airway maintenance portion of the initial assessment in pediatric trauma.

During the initial evaluation, identification of any foreign bodies, facial, mandibular, or tracheal fractures should be pursued with the initial physical exam. It is important to suction secretions and bleeding, and to position the head in a position that eliminates orophayngeal and pharyngeal obstruction. Jaw thrust maneuvers are usually safest when possible cervical injury has not been excluded. Patients with early GCS scores of less than eight should be intubated with a definitive airway. In certain instances, cerebral edema or traumatic fractures such as Leforte III fractures which can lead to cerebral edema will require control of the airway by intubation or creation of a surgical airway. If the patient's airway is initially stable and not affected by the traumatic injury or other causative elements, a reassessment of the airway should be continually repeated as deterioration could happen later.

Airway Evaluations

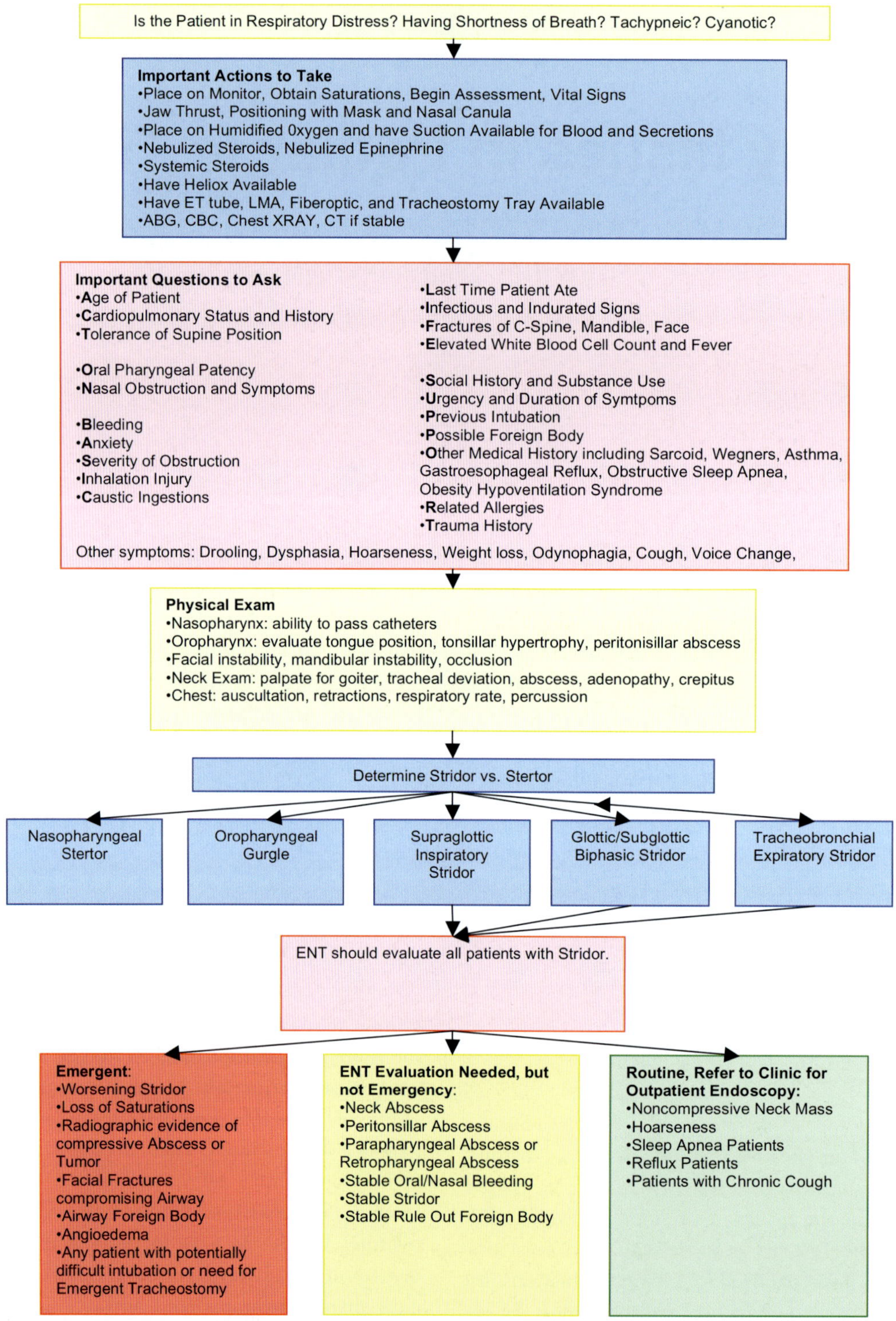

Fig 1–1. Algorithm for airway evaluation.

A difficult airway can be anticipated and preparation is the key for such events. If correct jaw thrust position is obtained, mask ventilation may be supported until an appropriate environment is created for a surgical airway.[2] New evidence supports the use of the LMA for children when there is difficulty in identification of the glottis on laryngoscopy.[3] All equipment for intubation and possible tracheotomy should be available to the primary responder while trying to establish a difficult airway.[4]

Children should be placed on oxygen during the initial assessment. An oral airway is advantageous only when a patient is unconscious. Nasopharyngeal airways can be used in the conscious patient. When the airway will require intubation, important decisions are determined as to which type of intubation. Nasotracheal intubation is preferred in a conscious patient with cervical spine injuries. This method is contraindicated in patients with extensive maxillofacial injuries. Orotracheal intubation is indicated for the trauma patient who has had significant head trauma requiring hyperventilation, a patient who cannot protect his or her airway due to collapse of soft tissue, secretions, or bleeding, and a child suffering from hypovolemia who will need to go to the operating room[5] (Fig 1–3).

Specifically, in children, it is important to remember some key anatomic differences in the initial trauma assessment. Pediatric patients have a greater size disproportion between the cranium and the midface. A child's airway is often protected from the known sniffing position seen by their slightly more superior and anterior midface. This is also a result, in part, due to the cricoid being located at the 4th cervical vertebra level rather than the adult 7th cervical vertebrae.

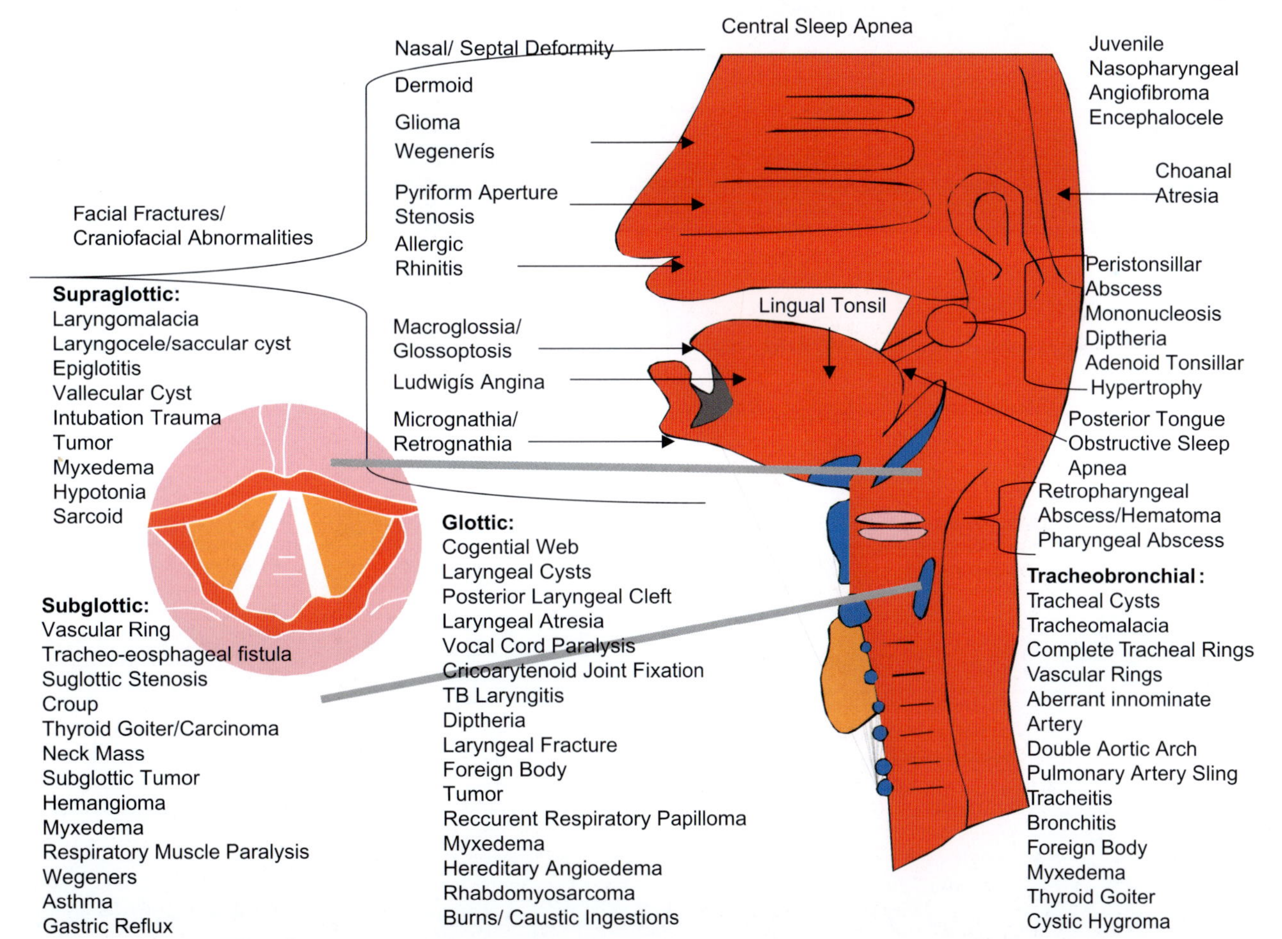

Fig 1–2. Differential diagnosis of airway obstruction by anatomic location.

Additional anatomic differences when compared to adults can make intubation of the pediatric patient challenging. The pediatric oropharynx tends to be disproportionately small when considering children's large tongue and tonsil size making laryngeal exposure on intubation difficult. The larynx itself is more anterior and lies higher than the adult larynx. Moreover, the infant larynx is approximately one-third the size of the adult larynx. The smaller size results in a significant reduction in the overall laryngeal airway. Pediatric patients have the smallest area in their airway at the level of the cricoid ring. The vocal cord is approximately 7 to 8 mm long. The subglottis measures 4.5 to 7 mm in diameter. Thus, if cricoid dimensions are less than 4 mm, the patent is considered to have subglottic stenosis. Another critical fact is that an infant's trachea is 5 cm long and grows to 7 cm by 18 months. This very short tracheal length should be recalled upon intubation to prevent mainsteming and inadequate ventilation.

Nasotracheal intubation is discouraged in patients under the age of 12. The blind passage of an endotracheal tube around the anterosuperior glottis makes this an extremely difficult intubation. It is also important to remember that even small amounts of swelling in the pediatric airway can contribute to marked stenosis and clinical stridor.[6]

When a patient has severe facial fractures, laryngotracheal trauma, or difficult intubation, a surgical airway is required (Fig 1–4). The four types of surgical airways include: tracheostomy, cricothyrotomy, needle cricothyrotomy, and percutaneous transtracheal ventilation. In the event that a surgical airway is needed, cricothyroidotomy should only be performed in patients greater than 11 years of age. Of the four methods to establish a surgical airway, needle cricothyrotomy is the preferred procedure for children.[7]

The key to providing an emergency airway is anticipation, preparation, and controlled attempts at resuscitation. The figures in this chapter demonstrate the plethora of possible causes of airway obstruction. In the workup of the pediatric trauma patient, it is vital to determine the source of obstruction. Once the cause of obstruction is diagnosed,

ALGORITHM 1
RAPID SEQUENCE INTUBATION (RSI)
FOR THE PEDIATRIC PATIENT

Preoxygenate

Atropine sulfate
0.1ñ0.5 mg

Sedation

Hypovolemic
Midazolam HCl 0.1 mg/kg
(5 mg maximum)

Normovolemic
Thiopental sodium
4ñ5 mg/kg

Cricoid Pressure

Paralysis*
Succinylcholine chloride
<10 kg: 2 mg/kg
>10 kg: 1 mg/kg

Intubate, Check Tube Position,
Release Cricoid Pressure

* Proceed according to clinical judgment and skill/experience level

Fig 1–3. Rapid sequence intubation for pediatric patients (Advanced Trauma Life Support, 2003.[4])

an appropriate treatment plan can be placed with proper backup equipment for possible need of a surgical airway. All services providing initial assessment should work together in a coordinated effort to provide a safe and stable environment for the patient. Once the airway is secured and the steps in the ABCDE algorithm are executed, attention can be turned to the facial fracture and traumatic injury.

REFERENCES

1. Lalwani A. *Current Diagnosis and Treatment in Otolaryngology- Head and Neck Surgery*. New York, McGraw-Hill; 2004:481–495.
2. Orenstein J. Prehospital pediatric airway management. *Clini Ped Emerg Med.* 2006:7:31–37.
3. Meyer R, Brambrink R, Ansgar M. Management of the paediatric airway: new developments. *Curr Opin Anaesthesiol.* 2002:15:329–337.
4. American College of Surgeons. *Advanced Trauma Life SupportforDoctors.* SeventhImpression.Chicago,Ill: 2003: 26–31.
5. Lore J, Medina J. *An Atlas of Head and Neck Surgery*. Philadelphia, Pa: Elsevier Saunders; 2005:82–85.
6. Pasha R. *Otolaryngology Head and Neck Surgery Clinical Reference Guide*. San Diego, Calif: Plural Publishing; 2006.
7. Bailey B, Calhoun K, Friedman N, Newlands S. *Head and Neck Surgery-Otolaryngology*. Philadelphia, Pa: Lippincott Williams; 2001:677–688.

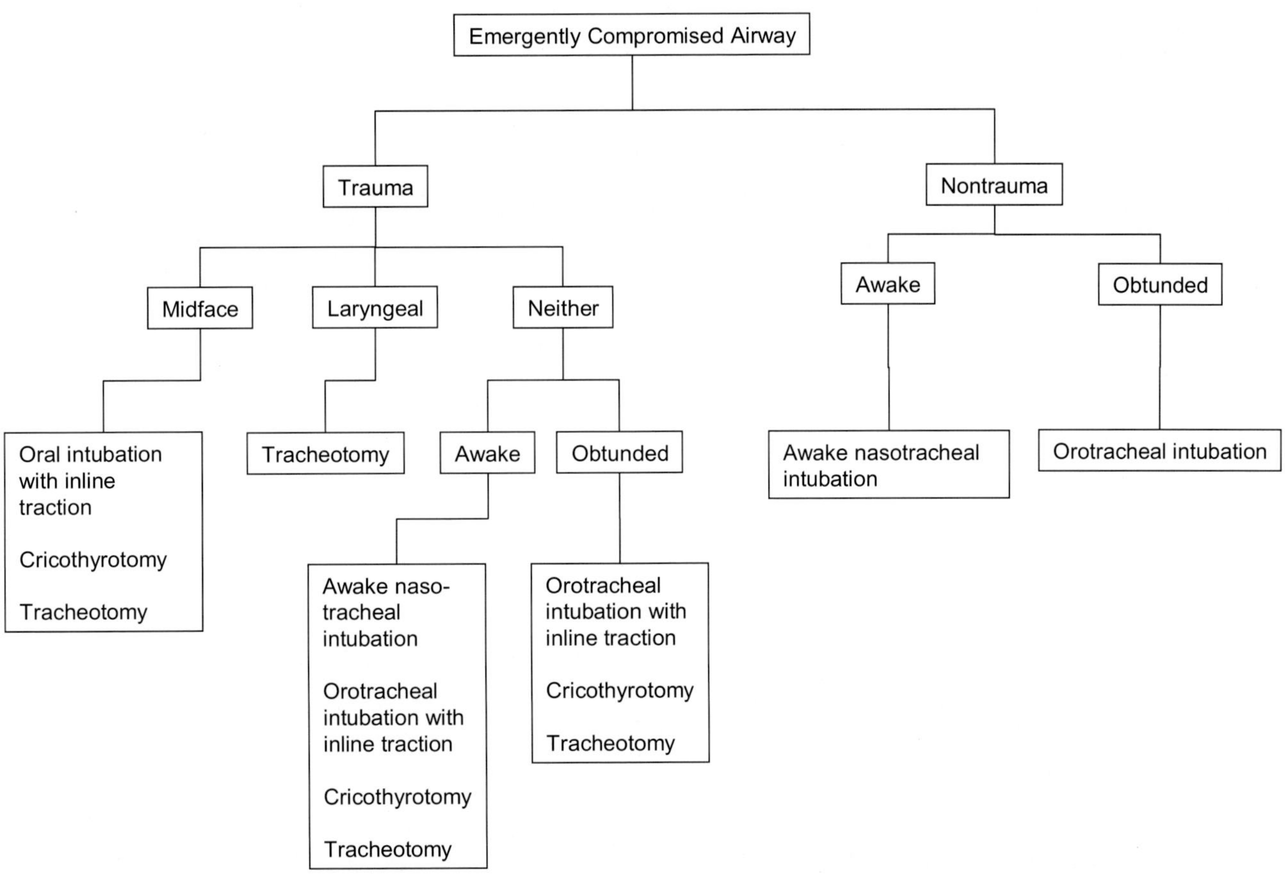

Fig 1–4. Emergency management of the airway (Bailey, 2001).[7]

2

Resorbable Materials in Pediatric Craniofacial Trauma Surgery

Martin B. Steed

Scientific advances in the field of biomaterials have continuously allowed surgeons the ability to improve craniofacial trauma patient care. The development of resorbable materials in the arena of craniofacial and trauma surgery lends itself especially well to the pediatric trauma patient population. Concerns of possible growth restriction or migration in pediatric patients who have titanium plates and screws placed within their facial and cranial skeleton have led surgeons to explore the use of bioabsorbable materials which could be designed to maintain favorable biomechanical properties to allow for adequate healing and then absorb without incident (Fig 2–1). Early difficulties in the use of these materials included localized inflammatory reactions and prolonged degradation times, but these have become less common with advances in the polymer choice and ratio of these polymers. Current research endeavors have focused on ascertaining the ability of the absorbable devices to withstand the functional demands of the pediatric maxillofacial skeleton and improving the technical aspects of placing the devices.

A great many of the significant contributions evaluating the use of resorbable materials in the pediatric craniofacial skeleton found the literature come from studies in craniofacial and orthognathic surgery in the pediatric skeleton. Technical biomechanical advances and successful in vivo studies have brought us to the point where the resorbable plating materials can be considered for a number of the varying types of pediatric craniofacial fractures (Figs 2–2 and 2–3). The use of resorbable plates and screws in the pediatric patient who has sustained a mandible fracture continues to be controversial and has received attention in the pediatric craniofacial literature in the recent past, mostly through the use of self-reinforced resorbable biomaterials.[1,2] These injuries have traditionally been treated with a short period of intermaxillary fixation

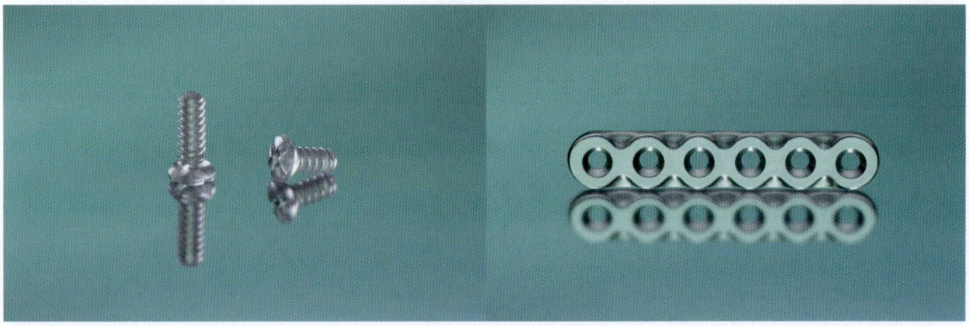

Fig 2-1. Resorbable screws and plate (Inion system).

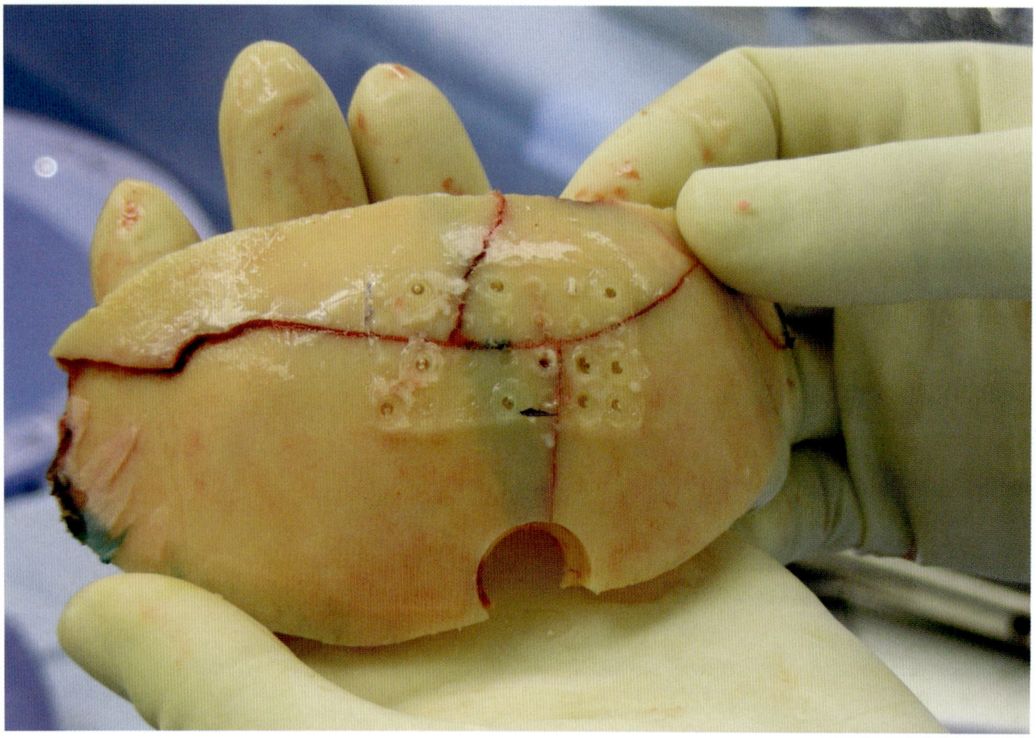

Fig 2–2. A resorbable sheet employed to reduce a frontal bone fracture after craniotomy.

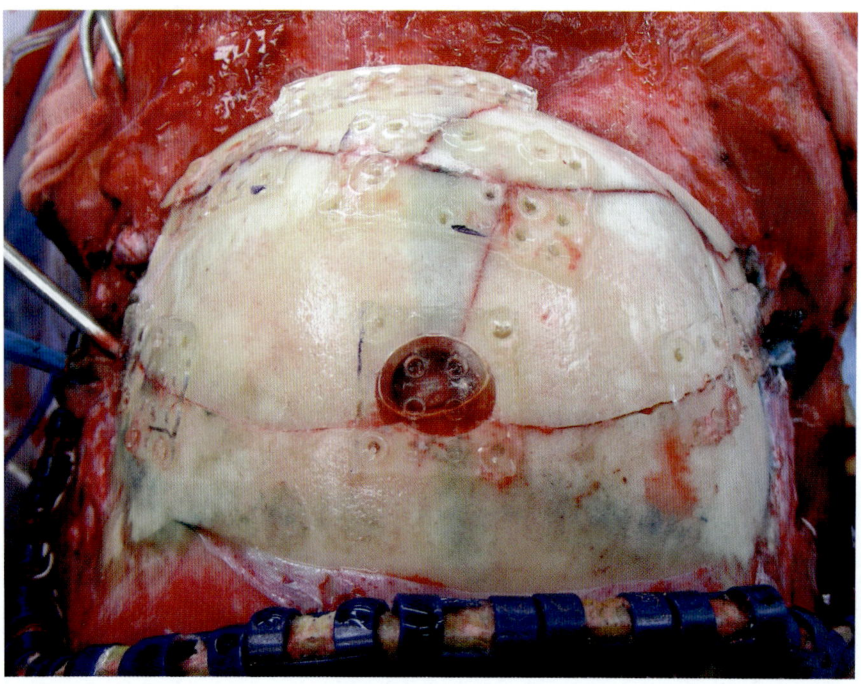

Fig 2–3. Resorbable sheets employed to fixate frontal bone fracture after craniotomy.

or through the use of guiding elastics secondary to the short period of time necessary for bony healing.

HISTORY OF RESORBABLE PLATING OF THE CRANIOFACIAL SKELETON

Synthetic bioabsorbable materials have been used for over four decades. They were first used as membranes and suture material in the form of resorbable sutures such as polyglycolic acid (Dexon), polyglyconate (Maxon), polyglycolic-poly-L-lactide copolymer (Vicryl), and polydioxanne (PDS). The experimental use of resorbable plates and screws were brought to the literature in the 1970s and the first clinical reports on the use of polylactic plates were published in the international literature in the 1980s.[3] The first reports were promising, but soon were followed by cases of long-term adverse reactions during resorption.[4]

Cutwright et al used resorbable materials (PLA suture) in the correction of mandible fractures in *Macaca* rhesus monkeys and performed histologic analysis of the healing sites in 1971.[5] One year later, Getter and Cutright et al used poly-L-lactide plates and screws for the treatment of mandibular fractures in six beagle dogs and by 32 to 40 weeks the fracture sites were indistinguishable from the adjacent bone.[6] The use of resorbable plates in the fixation of maxillofacial bone was initially reported in the literature by Kulkarni et al in 1971.[7] Pilot studies in the early 1970s concluded that the use of resorbable plates and screws in the maxillofacial skeleton were not mechanically adequate without intermaxillary fixation and were of excessive thickness for use in the craniofacial skeleton.

The inability to provide adequate strength with acceptable degradation time led to the development of systems incorporating a combination of the polylactic acid and polyglycolic acid materials in a varying ratio. The first resorbable plating system approved by the US Food and Drug Administration (FDA) for use in nonload-bearing areas of the craniofacial skeleton was in 1996 (82% polylactic and 18% polyglycolic acid [PLLA-PGA, LactoSorb®; Walter Lorenz Surgical, Jacksonville, Fla]). There are currently approximately eight systems available for use in the craniofacial skeleton in the United States.[8] Eppley et al first reported their experience and success with copolymer PLLA and PGA biodegradable materials for maxillofacial trauma, including Le Fort fractures, zygomaticomaxillary complex fractures, and orbital rim and floor fractures.[9]

The use of resorbable materials in the treatment of pediatric craniofacial trauma continues to gain clinical acceptance as demonstrated by larger studies with successful outcomes as demonstrated by Bell et al in 2006[10] in a retrospective analysis of a series of 59 patients and Eppley et al[11] in 2005 in a series of 44 patients.

Rigid metal fixation of mandibular fractures in children can be complicated by a mixed dentition that can occupy the entire vertical dimension of the bone and places teeth and the inferior alveolar nerve at risk during screw insertion. In addition, ongoing development of the mandible poses the potential risk of intrabony translocation of metal plates and screws, risking potential growth and teeth disturbances and difficulty with secondary removal if needed. The use of resorbable plating in the pediatric mandible will continue to be explored within the craniofacial trauma literature.

TITANIUM IMPERFECTIONS

Titanium plating systems have provided the surgeon treating craniofacial trauma the ability to rigidly fixate fractures with a biologically extremely well-tolerated and biomechanically strong material. The plates, screws, and mesh materials that are placed in adult trauma patients very often do not require removal after they have served their purpose and fracture healing is completed.

The placement of fixed nonresorbable plating systems in the immature and growing craniofacial skeleton of children and infants, however, has sparked much debate. Rigid fixation-induced growth restriction, hardware migration, and plate and screw fate are issues that remain unresolved as adequate data addressing each of these issues are limited.

Influence on Growth

Several animal studies have been conducted to examine the possible effects of rigid fixation on craniofacial growth. Growth disturbances have been observed with rigid plate fixation in rabbits when plates were placed across cranial sutures,[12-15] and they may occur even when suture lines are not crossed, as found by Yaremchuk et al[16] in monkeys. The impact of open reduction and internal fixation with titanium plates in pediatric trauma patients on facial growth remains unclear.

Migration of Plates and Screws

Migration of fixation devices is of particular concern in the pediatric cranium. It is known that miniplates and screws have the capacity to migrate in bone as well as other tissues such as cartilage. Growth of the skull takes place by the laying of new bone on the outer surface and resorption of old bone on the inner table. Plates and screws applied on the outer surface of the skull are occasionally found sunk in the bone or even on the inner side of the skull lying against the dura.[17,18] Hönig et al observed that total invagination of titanium plates with initial intracranial translocation occurred 12 to 16 weeks after implantation.[19]

Thermal Sensitivity

Although a somewhat uncommon complaint, thermal conductivity of titanium plates can be a postoperative concern of the patient. This could become especially problematic in colder climates with larger plates and minimal soft tissue coverage.

Interference with Future Imaging

Titanium plates do not allow full visualization of the fracture line on postoperative plain or panoramic radiographs. As resorbable plates are radiolucent, full visibility of the fracture site is available to the clinician. When resorbable plates or mesh is used to stabilize bone graft reconstruction of larger defects, the radiolucent property may enable the surgeon to see the progress of the bone graft easily.[20] Artifact is often encountered in postoperative computed tomography scans and/or magnetic resonance imaging when titanium plates and screws are employed. This becomes of great concern when obtaining these images for evaluation of local tumor recurrence.

Palpability

The presence of thin tissue covering a titanium plate may lead to a patient complaint of palpability of the material after healing has been completed, often resulting in a disruptive second procedure for removal of the often integrated plate.

Influence on Radiotherapy

In patients who undergo both surgical and radiation therapy for malignant tumors of the head and neck the presence of a titanium reconstruction plate within the path of the radiation field may have some effect. Reconstructive metal plates scatter therapeutic radiation and can significantly affect dosimetry, especially to tissue directly adjacent to the plate.[21] As a result, the area covered by the plate requires more complicated dosimetry schemes to provide adequate therapeutic irradiation.[21-23]

Need for Subsequent Removal

Orringer et al reviewed the reasons for hardware removal in a series of craniofacial patients and found that palpable or prominent hardware was the most common cause for removal followed by loosening of plates and screws, pain, infection, wound dehiscence, thermal sensitivity, and plate migration.[24]

TYPES AND CHARACTERISTICS OF POLYMERS AND COPOLYMERS

Throughout their evolution, bioabsorbable osteofixation devices have been made of polymers such as:

- Poly-L-lactide (PLLA)
- Polyglycolide (PGA)

Or their copolymers such as:

- Polylactide-coglycolide (PLGA)
- Poly–L/D–lactide (P (L/DL) LA)

A differentiation must be understood between homopolymers and copolymers. Homopolymers (eg, polylactide or polyglycolide) are composed of repeating identical units (monomers) that are derived from [alpha]-hydroxy acids. When two or more different monomers are used, a copolymer is formed (eg, PLGA or P (L/DL) LA). The ratio of the homopolymer used is usually denoted in a ratio form. For example, PLGA (85:15) denotes 85% polylactic acid and 15% polyglycolic acid.

Polylactide contains a methyl group (-CH_3) that makes polylactide more hydrophobic and thus more resistant to hydrolysis than polyglycolide. Polylactide that has been used in past clinical applications has commonly been pure poly-L-lactide. L-lactide polymers are semicrystalline and characterized by high strength and long degradation time whereas glycolide polymers are amorphous with lower strength, but rapid degradation time. In pure poly-L-lactide, the identical polymer chains can be tightly packed, which makes the polymer partly crystalline. Crystallinity and hydrophobicity make poly-L-lactide very resistant to hydrolysis and biodegradation.

The development of copolymers with varying ratios has attempted to optimize the plates and screws to maintain adequate strength while developing a favorable resorption profile with minimal local inflammation. Adding D-isomers into an L-isomer–based polymerization system results in winding polymer chains, which cannot be tightly packed.[25] Thus, P (L/DL) LA is amorphous and more susceptible to hydrolysis and biodegradation. The physical characteristics of the slowly degrading poly-L-lactide and the very rapidly degrading polyglycolide can be modified by the copolymerization of various proportions of homopolymers: 70/30 P (L/DL) LA is an example of this optimization; 70/30 P (L/DL) LA retains approximately 68% of its initial bending strength after 8 weeks, approximately 30% after 6 months, and is approximately 80% resorbed at 80 weeks.

Polymers exhibit a glass-transition temperature, above which the polymer is soft and malleable. The glass-transition temperature of poly-L-lactide is 57°C, and of polyglycolide, 36°C. This temperature needs to be reached to allow the contouring of the plate to allow proper adaptation to the fracture site.

Both lactic acid and glycolic acid are produced during normal cell metabolism. Lactic acid has two enatiomeric forms, L-lactide and D-lactic acid. The resorption process for PLA occurs in two phases:

1. *Hydrolysis:* Hydrolysis occurs when body fluids (water) enter the implant, chemically react with the polymer, and break down the polymer chains.
2. *Fragmental metabolization:* Fragmental metabolization occurs when the polymer continues to fragment until single lactic acid molecules are finally metabolized in the liver into carbon dioxide (CO_2) and water (H_2O) (Fig 2–4).

During the degradation process, the resorbable polymer converts into CO_2 and H_2O by the process of bulk hydrolysis and resorbs completely. The timing of this resorption is clinically of great importance and continues to be evaluated and modified with different ratios and types of polymers.

In 2001, Bos detailed the difficulties and clarified the differences between the assessment of bioresorption and biodegradation.[26] Bioresorption is the process of removal by cellular activity and/or dissolution of a material in a biologic environment. A material is considered resorbed once all molecules have been removed. Biodegradation is the process in which the gradual breakdown of a material is mediated by specific biologic activity. Biodegradation is the

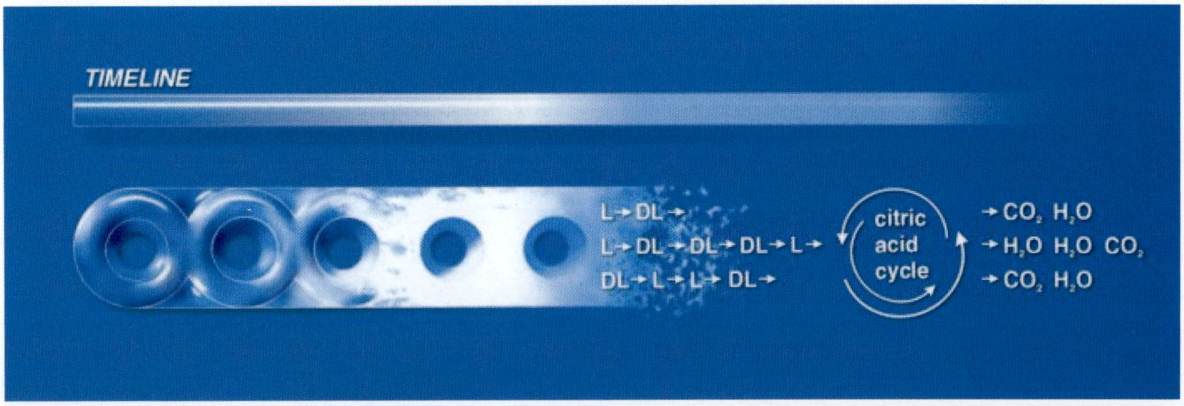

Fig 2–4. Fragmental metabolization.

body's way of "breaking down" a polymer whereas bioresorption is the body's way of "clearing out" the polymer.[8]

Various techniques have been used to facilitate polyglycolide, polylactide, or their copolymers into osteofixation devices. Melt molding usually produces devices that are either too brittle or too flexible for osteofixation. Compression molding or injection molding produces moderately strong devices.

The strength of biodegradable materials is usually achieved by the production of bulky and large devices to provide adequate stability. Professor Törmälä and Professor Rokkanen developed a self-reinforcing technique in 1988 in Finland.[21] This technique made it possible to manufacture strong devices for osteosynthesis in load-bearing bones. The bone plates could also be bent at room temperature, which made them easy to use. Ultra-high-strength (bending strength up to approximately 400 mega Pascal) self-reinforced implants can be developed by sintering and by solid-state deformation techniques. The self-reinforcement technique uses the solid-state deformation of a polymer material to yield a composite in which matrix and reinforcing elements are of the same polymer. Self-reinforced devices are superior in terms of mechanical strength and handling properties and can often be contoured below the glass transition temperature.

TECHNICAL PITFALLS

As with any new material and technique there is a learning curve for the surgeon placing resorbable plates and screws in the pediatric trauma patient. Two important intraoperative differences between titanium and the resorbable plates and screws remain. These are the need for a heating device to provide malleability and the need to tap the bone prior to screw placement. Care must be taken in placing the screws as excessive pressure upon tightening of the screws can result in the screw head shearing off. Many advocate that a second screw can be placed within the same location simply by redrilling through the previous screw, tapping, and placing another.

The resorbable plates available at present are bulkier than a titanium plate and placement can be difficult in comminuted fractures. The thin bone present along the maxilla and medial orbit makes tapping for screw placement difficult.

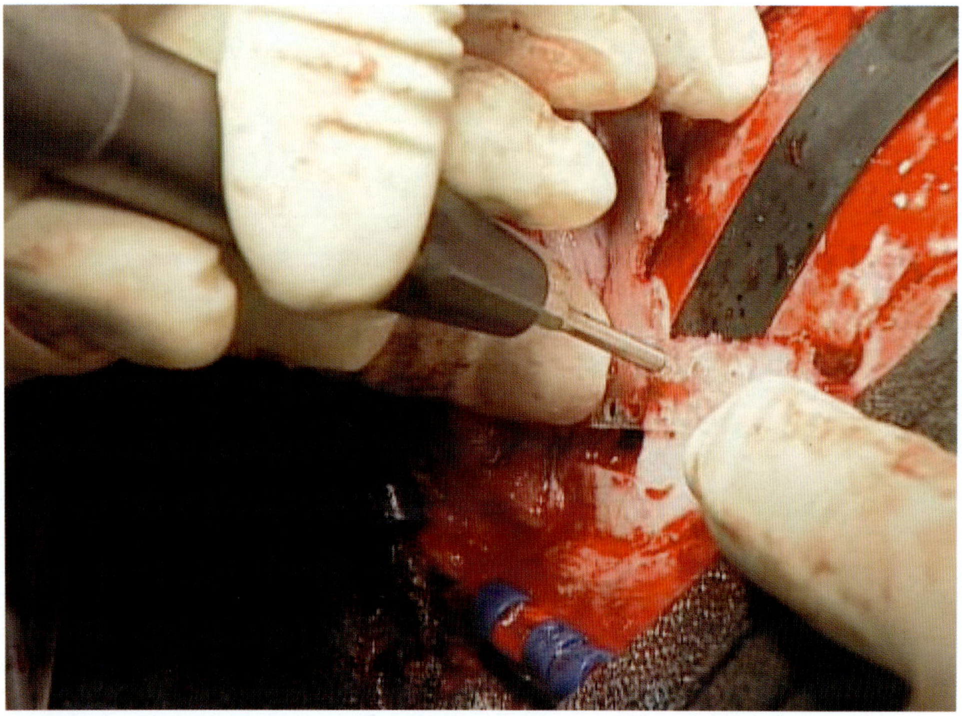

Fig 2–5. Placement of resorbable pin with KLS Martin Sonic Weld (SonicWeld Rx.).

Technical advances in placement of resorbable fixation such as the KLS ultrasonic pin-weld technology allows for placement of pins without the need for tapping and may make obtainment of fixation more straightforward (Fig 2–5). This technology utilizes ultrasound to melt the pin as it comes into contact with a hard surface such as bone.

COMPLICATIONS

Sterile Abscess Formation/Localized Inflammatory Response

The foreign body reaction seen with the use of resorbable materials is thought to result from the macrophage-mediated inflammatory response. This process can induce cell death and an acute inflammatory response that can become evident even after a considerable time has elapsed since implantation.[27] Such late adverse reactions caused by the implant degradation or host immunologic factors, or both, need further investigation.[28] Studies suggest that the mechanism of degradation varies between subcutaneous and intraosseous PLLA implants, and that the histological reaction induced by the implant may also vary.[27-29] A general hypothesis, based on the experience of several research groups, is that the tissue response to degrading polymer correlates with the relationship between local accumulation of polymer debris from degrading implants and the capacity of surrounding tissues to eliminate such debris, and with host buffer capacity and increased osmotic pressure.[28,29] This is thought to become clinically significant in cases where a rapidly resorptive material such as pure PGA is used or when a recipient patient is unable to resorb the material over a long period of time. The use of materials with amorphous (noncrystalline) composition has been the most significant advancement in this regard.

Load Bearing Areas—Pediatric Mandible

Yerit et al evaluated the use of SR materials in the fractured pediatric mandible in 2005.[2] Their study evaluated the stability and efficiency of biodegradable self-reinforced plates and screws in a series of 13 patients varying in age from 5 to 16 years who had sustained mandible fractures. They found that the self-reinforced devices provided sufficient rigidity and strength to allow for bony union to occur without the need for intermaxillary fixation except in the presence of a concurrent condylar process fracture. The authors state that the inferior border of the mandible is the best place for the positioning of a plate in these fracture sites. Angular fractures together with fractures of the ramus and the condyles can be internally fixed with miniplates or microplates, whereas the body of the mandible remains a complicated operation site due to close tooth buds in young children.[2] The presence of the permanent tooth buds makes positioning of the plate difficult and bicortical screw placement often impossible. One significant advantage of resorbable screws in the pediatric mandible is the avoidance of potential odontogenic injury. As the drill hole and tapping of the screw threads penetrate only the outer cortex, injury to developing teeth is unlikely.[11]

Despite these advances, further clinical outcomes support is likely to be needed before resorbable materials are embraced routinely by the majority of surgeons treating pediatric mandibular trauma.

CONCLUSION

The use and support for resorbable fixation devices has increased dramatically in the past 10 years. Resorbable plates and screws have been used successfully in the pediatric craniofacial skeleton within the craniofacial, orthognathic, and trauma arenas and their use will likely continue to increase as further clinical studies evaluate outcomes and complication rates.

REFERENCES

1. Ylikontiola L, Sundqvuist K, Sandor GK, Törmälä P, Ashammakhi N. Self-reinforced bioresorbable poly-L/DL-lactide [SRP(L/DL)LA] 70/30 miniplates and miniscrews are reliable for fixation of anterior mandibular fractures: a pilot study. *Oral Surg Oral Med Oral Pathol Oral Radiol Endod.* 2004;97:312–317.
2. Yerit KC, Hainich S, Enislidis G, et al. Biodegradable fixation of mandibular fractures in children: stability and early results. *Oral Surg Oral Med Oral Pathol Oral Radiol Endod.* 2005;100:17–24.

3. Suuronen R, Kontio R, Ashammakhi N, Lindqvist C, Laine, P. Bioabsorbable self-inforced plates and screws in craniomaxillofacial surgery. *Bio-Med Mater Engineer. 2004;14(4):*517–524.
4. Bergsma JE, Rozema FR, Bos RRM, De Bruijn WC. Foreign body reactions to resorbable poly (L-lactide) bone plates and screws used for the fixation of unstable zygomatic fractures. *J. Oral Maxillofac. Surg.*1993; 51:666–670.
5. Cutwright DE, Hunsuck E, Beasley JD. Fracture reduction using a biodegradable material, polylactic acid. *J Oral Surg.*1971;29:393–397.
6. Getter L, Cutwright DE, Bhaskar S, Augsburg J. A biodegradable intraosseous appliance in the treatment of mandibular fractures. *J Oral Surg.* 1972;30:344–348.
7. Kulkarni RK, Moore EG, Hegyeli AF, et al. Biodegradable poly (lactic acid) polymers. *J Biomed Mater Res.* 1971;5:169.
8. Ricalde P, Posnick JC. Degradation rate of delta (resorbable) internal fixation: report of 2 cases. *J Oral Maxillofac Surg.* 2004;62:250–255.
9. Eppley BL, Prevel CD. Nonmetallic fixation in traumatic midfacial fractures. *J Craniofac Surg.* 1997;8:103.
10. Bell RB, Kindsfater CS. The use of biodegradable plates and screws to stabilize facial fractures. *J Oral Maxillofac Surg.* 2006;64:31–39.
11. Eppley BL. Use of resorbable plates and screws in pediatric facial fractures. *J Oral Maxillofac Surg.* 2005;63:385–391.
12. Antikainen T, Pernu H, Törmälä P, et al. Development of the neurocranium after transsutural fixing by new, resorbable poly-L-lactide miniplates. A comparison to fixing with the common titanium miniplates. *Acta Neurochir (Wien).* 1994;128:26–31.
13. Resnick JI, Kinney BM, Kawamoto HK Jr. The effect of rigid internal fixation on cranial growth. *Ann Plast Surg.* 1990;25:372–374.
14. Wong L, Dufresne CR, Richtsmeier JT, et al. The effect of rigid fixation on growth of the neurocranium. *Plast Reconstr Surg.* 1991;88:395–403.
15. Wong L, Richtsmeier JT, Manson PN. Craniofacial growth following rigid fixation: suture excision, miniplating, and microplating. *J Craniofac Surg.* 1993;4:234–244.
16. Yaremchuk MJ, Fiala TGS, Barker F, et al. The effect of rigid fixation on craniofacial growth in rhesus monkeys. *Plast Reconstr Surg.* 1994;93:1–15.
17. Fearon JA, Munro IR, Bruce DA. Observations on the use of rigid fixation for craniofacial deformities in infants and young children. *Plast Reconstr Surg.* 1995;95:634–637.
18. Papay FA, Hardy S, Morales Jr, L, et al. "False" migration of rigid fixation appliances in pediatric craniofacial surgery. *J Craniofac Surg.* 1995;6:309–313.
19. Hönig JF, Merten HA, Luhr HG. Passive and active intracranial translocation of osteosynthesis plates in adolescent minipigs. *J Craniofac Surg.* 1995;6:292–298.
20. Laughlin RM, Block MS, Wilk R, Malloy RB, Kent JN. Resorbable plates for mandibular fractures. *J Oral Maxillofac Surg.* 2007;65:89–96.
21. Scher N, Poe D, Kuchnir F, Reft C, Weichselbaum R, Panje WR. Radiotherapy of the resected mandible following stainless steel fixation. *Laryngoscope.* 1988;98:561–563.
22. Castillo MH, Button TM, Doerr R, Homs MI, Pruett CW, Pearce JI. Effects of radiotherapy on mandibular reconstruction plates. *Am J Surg.* 1988;156:261–263.
23. Gullane PJ. Primary mandibular reconstruction: analysis of 64 cases and evaluation of interface radiation dosimetry on bridging plates. *Laryngoscope.* 1991;101:1–24.
24. Orringer JS. Barcelona V. Buchman SR. Reasons for removal of rigid internal fixation devices in craniofacial surgery. *J Craniofac Surg.* 1998;9:40–44.
25. Kallela I, Tulamo RM, Hietanen J, Pohjonen T, Suuronen R, Lindqvist C. Fixation of mandibular body osteotomies using biodegradable amorphous self-reinforced (70L:30DL) polylactide or metal lag screws: an experimental study in sheep. *J Cranio-Maxillofac Surg.* 1999;27, 124–133.
26. Bos RR. Discussion: the fate of resorbable poly-L-lactic/polyglycolic acid (LactoSorb) bone fixation devices in orthognathic surgery. *J Oral Maxillofac Surg.* 2001;59:19–25.
27. Bergsma EJ, Rozema FR, Bos RRM, et al. In vivo degradation and biocompatibility study of in vitro predegraded as polymerized polylactide particles. *Biomaterials.* 1995; 16:267–274.
28. Suuronen R, Pohjonen T, Hietanen J, et al. A 5-year in vitro and in vivo study of the biodegradation of polylactide plates. *J Oral Maxillofac Surg.* 1998;56:604.
29. Van der Elst M, Kuiper I, Klein CPAT, et al. The burst phenomenon, an animal model simulating the long-term tissue response on PLLA interlocking nails. *J Biomed Mater Res.* 1996;30:139–143.

3

Soft Tissue and Bony Injury of the Pediatric Face

Russell Ashinoff
Albert Losken

INTRODUCTION

Maxillofacial injuries are among the most common reasons for childhood emergency room visits. Although rarely life threatening, there are numerous considerations that must be taken into account when evaluating young patients.

The approach to the pediatric maxillofacial trauma patient is somewhat different from the approach to the adult patient. Children are normally apprehensive in the hospital environment, especially after an injury, and are less likely to be able to communicate their complaints. Additionally, the possibility of abuse exists and must be considered as part of the workup.

ASSESSMENT AND DIAGNOSIS

The initial assessment and management of patients who present with maxillofacial trauma proceeds according to Advanced Trauma Life Support guidelines. The facial injuries are only considered after the "ABCDE"s (Airway, Breathing, Circulation, Disability, Exposure) of ATLS are evaluated and life-threatening injuries are addressed. Cervical spine injuries are common in patients who have sustained maxillofacial trauma and therefore must be given the appropriate consideration.[1]

The physical exam of the face begins with a systematic inspection and palpation beginning at the scalp and proceeding to the clavicles. The cranium, frontal bones, orbits, zygomatic arch, maxilla, and mandible are palpated. Obvious deformities, edema, hematoma, ecchymosis, and lacerations are noted. An exam of the oral cavity, the internal nose, and the external auditory canal is mandatory. The lacrimal apparatus, the parotid duct, and the facial nerve branches must be evaluated if the injury is near these structures. Lacerations are probed with a gloved finger to evaluate for bony deformities. If the patient is conscious and cooperative, sensory and motor function of the face is also evaluated.

Radiologic exams are important tools in the diagnosis of facial fractures. CT scanning with direct or reconstructed coronal images is the current standard of care and provides increased diagnostic accuracy over conventional radiographs.

Orbits

Inspect the palpebral fissures and height of the medial and lateral canthi on both sides. Palpate the rim for crepitus, tenderness, or step-offs. The globe is inspected for subconjunctival hemorrhage, proptosis, and enophthalmos. The pupils are evaluated for direct and indirect stimulation to light. If the patient is old enough, visual fields, visual acuity, and diplopia are determined, as is sensation in the distribution of the infraorbital nerve. The extraocular movements are evaluated. If the patient is comatose, a forced duction test is performed. Ophthalmologic consultation is appropriate when injuries involve the structures of the orbit.

Zygoma and Zygomatic Arch

Injuries to the zygoma and arch commonly occur in conjunction with orbital injuries; therefore, the evaluation of these structures should also include an orbital examination. The malar eminence should be examined from above to determine if flattening is present and should be palpated for step-offs. Limited mandibular excursion or pain (trismus) may indicate a zygomatic arch fracture. Sensation in the infraorbital nerve distribution should be assessed if possible.

Nose

The external nose is evaluated for deformity, swelling, ecchymosis, and epistaxis. An internal nasal exam is mandatory to evaluate the septum for deformity or hematoma. The initial assessment requires a higher index of suspicion because of the dissipation of forces that may cause a diffuse edema and make a fracture difficult to identify on physical exam.

SOFT TISSUE INJURIES

The initial exam should proceed as described previously, paying particular attention to critical structures that may be involved, such as the lacrimal apparatus, parotid duct, or facial nerve. Sedation is often necessary for the exam and/or the repair. Adequate anesthesia and physical restraint is a less desirable alternative.

Anesthetic choices include LET (Lidocaine 4%, Epinephrine 1:2000, Tetracaine 0.5–1%), which is combined with methylcellulose gel and applied to the wound for 15 to 45 minutes prior to manipulation. This often obviates the need for injection, but there are drawbacks. Due to concerns of systemic toxicity and difficulty of application, it is not recommended for use on mucosal surfaces. The vasoconstrictve effect may obscure important landmarks, for example,the vermilion border. Because of this, it is important to mark these structures in advance or consider an alternative method. Local infiltration with lidocaine, with or without epinephrine is a second option. Epinephrine should be avoided in terminal structures, such as the earlobe or nasal tip. Bicarbonate may be added to the lidocaine as a buffer to increase the pH and decrease the burning sensation experienced. This should be injected with a small needle (30-g). A regional block can also be used where appropriate, such as the lip or the ear.

Sedation is often coordinated by the ER physician and can range from moderate with a combination of Tylenol with codeine and oral versed to deep sedation with intravenous ketamine. Many other options exist and are beyond the scope of this discussion.

Once the patient is adequately anesthetized, the wound should be inspected. A copious amount of normal saline should be used to irrigate the wound thoroughly. Foreign bodies should be removed and the wound edges should be conservatively debrided. The goal of the repair is a precise approximation of wound edges and a layered, tension-free closure. It may be necessary to undermine the skin in the subcutaneous plane to accomplish this.

The skin is usually closed in two layers. The deep sutures serve to decrease tension and evert the wound edges. The superficial layer aligns the skin edges precisely and can be accomplished with Dermabond or suture. Although there are many suture options, general guidelines include absorbable suture (4-0 or 5-0 Monocryl or Vicryl) in the deep layer. The skin closure is accomplished with a fine absorbable suture (5-0 or 6-0 Fast Gut) in young children to avoid the trauma of suture removal. In older children, a fine nonabsorbable suture (5-0 or 6-0 nylon or Prolene) that is removed in 3 to5 days is appropriate. Mucosal surfaces are reapproximated with 4-0 or 5-0 chromic suture. Suture techniques include simple in an interrupted or running fashion, subcuticular, and mattress sutures. Care must be taken to make the simple sutures wider at the base of the repair to evert the skin and prevent dead space formation. Dermabond is appropriate in hairless areas, and should not be used on mucosal surfaces. Certain principles apply when closing facial lacerations on the face, and vary by location (Fig 3–1).

FOREHEAD

When repairing a forehead laceration it is important to approximate the deep layers of the wound to avoid

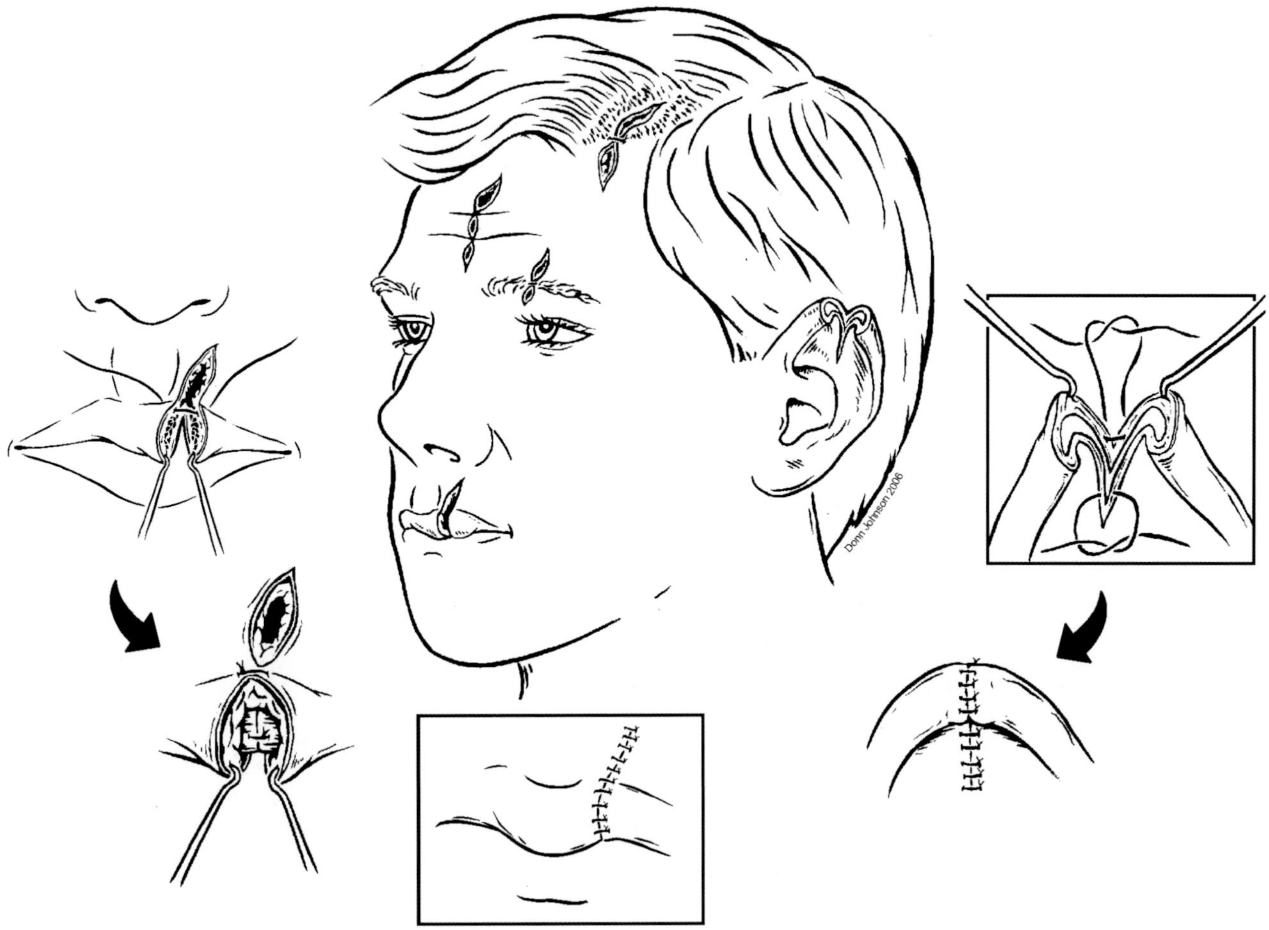

Fig 3-1. Principles of repair of facial lacerations.

a depressed scar. The hairline and skin creases must be precisely aligned to prevent noticeable deformities. If permanent suture is used, it should be removed in 3 to 5 days.

EYELID

Eyelid repairs in the emergency room usually require deep sedation. The surgeon must be aware of the possibility of concomitant ocular injuries and obtain an ophthalmologic consult if necessary. The lacrimal apparatus, medial, and lateral canthi must be evaluated and repaired if involved. This usually requires general anesthesia and is best accomplished in the operating room. A simple horizontal lid laceration can be repaired in a single layer, encompassing the skin and obicularis oculi muscle; 6-0 or 7-0 suture is normally used. Loupe magnification can be very helpful when repairing lid lacerations.

NOSE

It is important to determine if a septal hematoma is present and drain it. If the mucosa is lacerated, it is repaired with a 4-0 or 5-0 chromic or similar suture. The skin is repaired as described earlier. The alar margin, if involved, must be aligned precisely. It is not usually necessary to repair the cartilage, as the surrounding tissues hold it in place as it heals.

LIPS

When repairing lacerations of the lips it is important to align the anatomic landmarks precisely. For this reason, a regional block of the infraorbital and/or the mental nerve should be considered to avoid distortion of these landmarks. The vermilion border and the wet-dry border should be aligned before the remainder of the laceration is repaired. To avoid notching, vertical mattress sutures are used on the lip. If the obicularis oris is involved, it should be repaired with absorbable suture.

EARS

Regional block is useful for repairing laceration of the ear. The concha and external auditory canal are not anesthetized with this technique and must be infiltrated. Debridement should be avoided and cartilage should be preserved if possible. The skin closure will usually support the cartilage; rarely, an absorbable suture is necessary to repair the cartilage. A gauze bolster may be helpful to prevent hematoma.

FACIAL FRACTURES

The most common causes of facial fractures in the pediatric age group are falls and motor vehicle collisions. In children the fractures most often encountered are dentoalveolar fractures (34%) followed by zygoma fractures (30%) and Le Fort fractures (20%).

There are several differences in the anatomy of the pediatric craniofacial skeleton that contribute to the different fracture patterns seen in children. Children have a high cranial to facial volume ratio that decreases with increasing age. The face is retruded relative to the skull, which contributes to the predominance of cranial fractures and lower incidence of maxillary and midface fractures in younger children. As the ratio decreases, an increase in the predominance of facial fractures occurs. Flexible bone and suture lines, abundant adipose tissue, lack of sinus pneumatization, and the presence of tooth buds are other features that differentiate pediatric from adult fracture characteristics.

When treating pediatric facial fractures, the possibility of future growth disturbances must be considered. This is especially important when dealing with nasal septal injuries and condylar fractures.

The goal in the treatment of facial fractures in children, as in adults, is anatomic reduction of fractures and restoration of class I occlusion. Nondisplaced fractures can often be treated by observation, soft diet, and pain control. Displaced fractures require closed or open reduction and fixation with mandibulomaxillary fixation and/or internal plates and screws. Open reduction and internal fixation allows for stable reduction, primary bone healing, and decreases the need for, or duration of, mandibulomaxillary fixation. To minimize the possibility of future growth disturbance, subperiosteal dissection should be minimized and plates should not cross suture lines or the midline of the mandible. Hardware should be resorbable or removed as early as 2 to 3 months after placement, if permanent. Patients with open fractures should be treated with IV antibiotics.[2]

FRONTAL BONE FRACTURES

The frontal sinus develops at age 6 years and reaches adult size by late puberty. Prior to frontal sinus development, fractures tend to extend superiorly up the skull or across the orbital roof. Frontal sinus fractures in children are managed as those in adults. Fractures involving the posterior wall of the frontal sinus require a combined neurosurgical approach. After repair of any dural injuries, reduction and fixation of the bone fragments is performed. Autogenous cranial bone (full or split) can be used to span large bony defects or areas of comminution. If the sinus mucosa is severely disrupted, it should be obliterated and the frontonasal duct patency will need to be preserved with a catheter to prevent mucocele formation. Postoperatively, it is important to be alert for signs of a CSF leak.[3]

NASAL FRACTURES

The pediatric nose differs in a number of important aspects from that of an adult. It is composed largely of cartilage and bends easily during blunt trauma. In addition, the pediatric nose projects less than the adult nose. These factors contribute to the larger fracture segments and the higher incidence of septal hematoma seen in children. Nasal fractures can be purely bony (superior), purely cartilaginous (inferior), or a combination of the two. Diagnosis is usually based on physical exam, but CT is often obtained to rule out other fractures. As stated earlier, an intranasal exam is mandatory to rule out septal hematoma. The nasal septum is a major growth center which propels the maxilla downward and forward. A missed septal hematoma can result in septal necrosis and loss of support, leading to a saddle-shaped deformity. If discovered, a septal hematoma should be drained promptly.

The treatment of nasal fractures depends on the degree of displacement. Nondisplaced fractures can be observed. Displaced fractures should be reduced in a closed fashion within 3 to 7 days in children. Open reduction is to be avoided in children. Once anatomic reduction is achieved, intranasal packing or splinting for 3 days and external splinting for 7 days is performed. As swelling decreases, the external splint may need to be reapplied. Antibiotic coverage should be instituted if the packing remains for more than 24 hours.[3]

ORBITAL FRACTURES

Orbital fractures can be isolated or occur in conjunction with more complex fractures. The evaluation should include ophthalmologic evaluation and CT scan with coronal and axial sections (Fig 3–2). Operative intervention is indicated when comminuted fractures are present, and in cases of aesthetic or functional impairment. The goal is early treatment of soft tissue entrapment and restoration of orbital volume. Late management of diplopia and enophthalmos is difficult.

Orbital fractures are approached via a subciliary, transconjunctival, or infraorbital incision. Orbital floor fractures with large bony defects may require primary reconstruction with calvarial or rib grafts or, alternatively, resorbable plating systems. Comminuted orbital roof fractures may require a combined neurosurgical approach.[2]

NASO-ORBITOETHMOID FRACTURES (NOE)

These fractures are relatively uncommon in children. The naso-orbitoethmoid complex is defined anteriorly by the frontal process of the maxilla, the nasal process, and the spine of the frontal bone. Laterally, it is formed by the

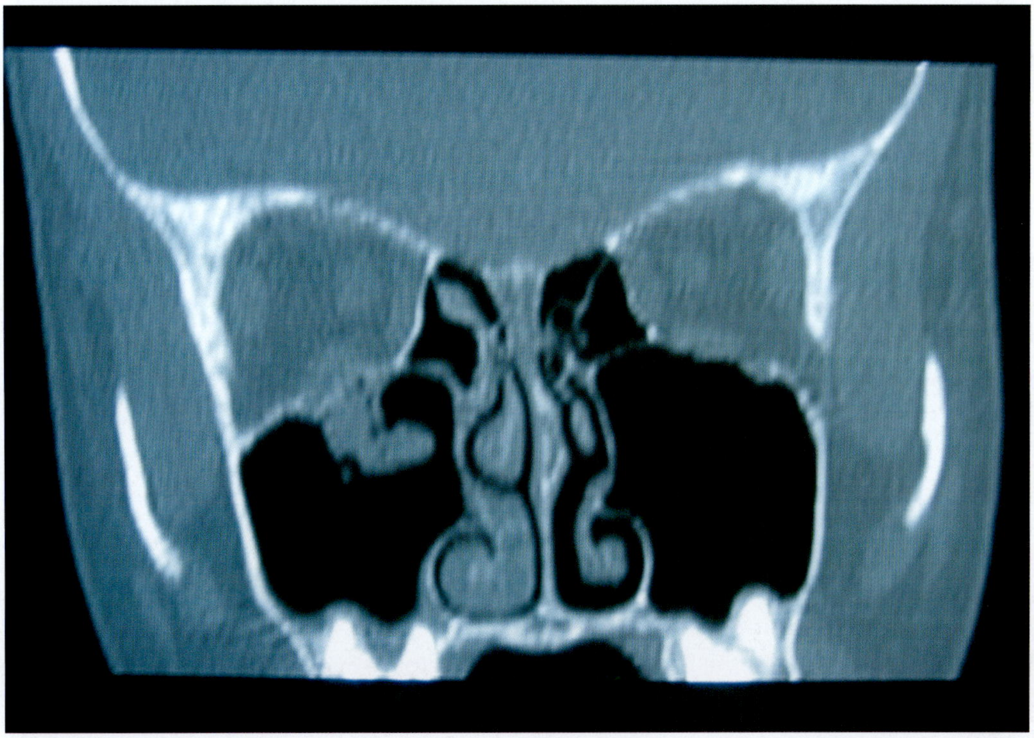

Fig 3-2. Coronal CT scan showing a right orbital floor fracture with soft tissue herniation in a patient with clinical entrapment.

lamina papyraceae and lacrimal fossae, and inferiorly by the ethmoidal labyrinths. Clinically, these patients have a flattened nose due to loss of nasal support and swollen medial canthal region, which may mask a traumatic telecanthus. Inability to pull the lower eyelid taut in a lateral direction usually indicates disruption of the medial canthal tendon. Nasal septal hematoma and dural tears on the region of the cribriform plate can also occur with this type of injury.

The treatment of NOE fractures in children is similar to that of adults and may require a combined neurosurgical approach. A coronal approach is utilized. After the neurosurgical team addresses brain injuries and dural tears, treatment consists of reduction and internal fixation of the larger bony segments. Nasal and orbital fractures are addressed individually. Care is taken to leave space for the nasal plate. The detached medial canthal tendon is usually attached to a bone fragment and must be repositioned and fixed with microplates or transnasal wires. Direct medial canthopexy is a last resort and often results in an unnatural appearance. When performed, it is important to pull the canthal tendon to a point behind the apex of the lacrimal fossa.[1,4]

ZYGOMATIC COMPLEX FRACTURES (ZMC)

Zygomatic complex fractures parallel the pneumatization of the maxillary sinus and are rare before 5 years of age. The zygoma articulates with the body of the sphenoid, frontal, and temporal bones and maxilla, forming a "tetrapod." These suture lines do not ossify until the seventh year of life. Most ZMC fractures actually represent a separation of the zygoma from adjacent bones either at the suture lines or by fractures of the other bones (Fig 3–3). These fractures tend to affect globe position because the zygoma forms a large part of the lateral orbital wall and floor. Signs and symptoms of these fractures may include enophthalmos, numbness in the infraorbital nerve distribution, diplopia, and trismus.

Nondisplaced fractures with no functional impairment may be treated with a soft diet and analgesics. Open treatment with fixation is indicated in comminuted fractures and in patients with functional impairment or aesthetic deformity. Treatment should commence within 3 to 5 days of the injury, as delay may increase the incidence of enophthalmos and the need for revisional surgery. The orbital floor, and zygomaticomaxillary and zygomaticofrontal buttresses should always be explored. Multiple incisions are used to reach the individual suture lines. A lateral eyebrow incision is used to access the zygomaticofrontal suture. The infraorbital rim and orbital floor are reached via a subciliary, transconjunctival, or infraorbital incision. The zygomaticomaxillary buttress is approached with a transoral buccal sulcus incision. In children, one-point fixation at the zygomaticofrontal suture may be adequate because of the shorter lever-arm action from the zygomaticofrontal suture to the infraorbital rim. Plating at the zygomatic buttress risks trauma to the maxillary tooth buds, especially in children under 6 years old.

Isolated, depressed, noncomminuted zygomatic arch fractures can be reduced with a Gillies temporal approach or buccal sulcus approach and are usually stable without fixation. Special situations include NOE and Le Fort III fractures. In these cases, the arch is approached via a coronal incision and rigidly fixed to restore facial width.[3]

LE FORT FRACTURES

Three types of Le Fort fractures have been defined. The Le Fort I fracture pattern is a horizontal maxillary fractrue. The Le Fort II pattern is a pyramidal midface fracture. The Le Fort III pattern is a craniofacial disarticulation. The goal of treatment is to restore facial height and projection. Isolated Le Fort I fractures usually can be treated with closed reduction and mandibulomaxillary fixation. Displaced fractures of the midface are treated with open reduction and internal fixation when it is possible to avoid damage to developing teeth. Reconstruction proceeds from inferior to superior. Otherwise, it may be necessary to utilize mandibulomaxillary fixation and suspension from the zygomatic arch for 2 to 3 weeks after the injury. Grossly comminuted fractures may need to be treated with a head frame that provides anterior traction.[5,3]

REFERENCES

1. American College of Surgeons. *Advanced Trauma Life Support Manual.* Chicago, Ill:2004.

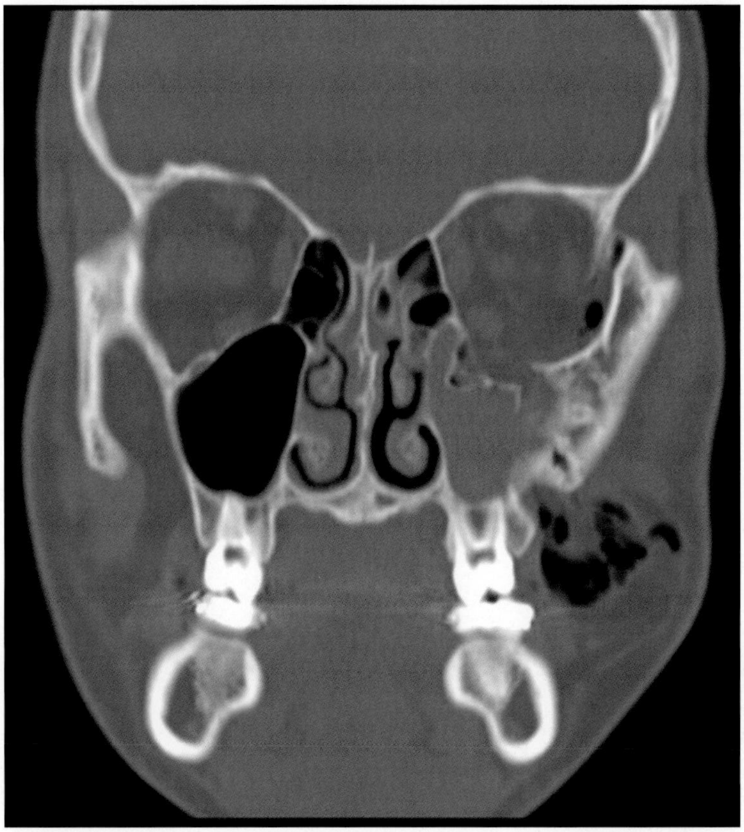

Fig 3-3. Coronal CT scan of a 16-year-old boy with a displaced left ZMC fracture.

2. Zimmermann CE, Troulis MJ, Kaban LB. Pediatric facial fractures: recent advances in prevention, diagnosis and management. *Int J Oral Maxillofac Surg.* 2006; 35(1):2–13.
3. Jones TR. Basic evaluation and management of maxillofacial trauma. In: Greco R.J. *Emergency Plastic Surgery.* Boston, Mass: Little Brown; 1991;285.
4. Hollier L, Thornton J. Facial fractures I: Upper two-thirds. *Select ReadPlast Surg.* 2002;9(26):1–34.
5. Thornton J, Hollier L, Facial fractures II: Lower third. *Select Read Plast Surg.* 2002;9(27):1–34.

4

Pediatric Orbital Trauma

C. Robert Bernardino

THE TRAUMA GAME

Children with facial trauma often have multiple injuries including ocular, neurosurgical, craniofacial, and systemic injuries. Although clinicians who manage facial trauma are often transfixed on the presence of ocular injuries, we must always focus on the proper order of managing injuries to save lives and minimize morbidity during recovery. Therefore, although ocular injuries may be present in a patient with craniofacial injury, we must ensure that, following the dictums of trauma management, we address first airway, breathing, and circulation issues prior to ocular issues. However, once a patient's emergency systemic issues are addressed, a patient with periocular trauma should be evaluated for vision-threatening trauma. Timely identification of vision-threatening trauma will allow for rapid repair and restoration of vision and the avoidance of worsening the ocular vision from other facial trauma rehabilitative surgery.

RUPTURED GLOBE

Probably the most important ocular injury to recognize is a ruptured globe. A ruptured globe is a full-thickness injury through the outer layers of the eye—the cornea and/or the sclera. As the eye is a pressurized organ, a rupture through the eye causes loss of internal pressure and allows internal vital structures of the eye to sublux outward. Also, with violation of the outer ocular shell, the risk for infection is high. In either case, damage to vital ocular structures can lead to permanent vision loss. Therefore, the identification of a ruptured globe is essential in managing periocular trauma.

Although a ruptured globe is often difficult to identify, the goal of a clinician is to determine if there is a high likelihood that a rupture is present, necessitating surgical exploration and possible repair. There are a number of different signs and symptoms patients may exhibit in the presence of a ruptured globe. The first sign is the presence of periocular trauma, particularly lacerating trauma. When a periocular laceration is present, one must be highly suspicious for a corneal or scleral laceration (Fig 4–1). If a laceration is present, one should carefully pull apart the eyelids to examine the eyeball (Fig 4–2); often the eyelids will be swollen or the patient will be guarding, making this difficult. Care also should be taken not to place pressure on the eyeball during examination; such pressure may worsen a ruptured globe, or unseal a self-sealing laceration.

Once the eyelids are opened, the eye should be examined in a systematic fashion, focusing on anterior structures first and then working deeper into the eyeball structures. Use of a hand-held penlight is useful to examine the eye. The cornea should be clear and have a crisp light reflex. Distortion of either may suggest the presence of a laceration, particularly if intraocular contents such as the iris are protruding through the laceration. The conjunctiva should also be assessed for chemosis (edema) or subconjunctival hemorrhage; the presence of either, particularly if focal, may represent an underlying laceration in the sclera.

Then the space between the cornea and the iris, the anterior chamber, should be examined. Normally, the anterior chamber should be clear and have a standard depth. If the depth is different, deeper or shallower, compared to the unaffected, contralateral side, the presence of a ruptured globe may be entertained. Also, the presence of blood, called a hyphema, is a sign of the presence of significant intraocular trauma including a ruptured globe. Even after a ruptured globe has been ruled out, a hyphema is a relative contraindication to periocular surgery (ie, fracture repairs) until it resolves. If one does not wait until resolution, a rebleed can occur causing increase in intraocular pressure and subsequent vision loss (glaucoma).[1]

The iris and, in particular, the pupil should be of its regular, round configuration. Distortion of the pupil's shape may suggest a rupture, particularly if it is teardrop shaped; the point of the teardrop may point at the rupture.

In examining a patient with periocular trauma, it is also important to check visual function. Visual acuity can be assessed with a traditional reading card or chart or, if unavailable, with any reading source such as a newspaper or other text. Vision should be checked on each eye individually, with the patient's spectacle correction if available. In the presence of a ruptured globe, vision is often depressed but not absolutely. If a patient cannot read in one eye, check for finger-counting vision, or if worse, hand-motion vision or light-perception vision.

Pupil reactivity also should be evaluated as it can be diminished in trauma to the eye. First, each pupil should be evaluated individually for its reaction to light, focusing on its briskness in constricting. A pupil that is sluggish to constrict may be a sign of significant intraocular injury. The light source should then be swung from one eye to another to evaluate both afferent and efferent function of the optic nerve. If a light source is swung from one eye to another (swinging penlight test) and the pupil dilates when the light is directly on it, but constricts when the light is on the contralateral side, then the afferent function of that side is compromised pointing to significant ocular or optic nerve injury.

Imaging studies often are helpful to determine if significant ocular trauma, in particular a ruptured globe, is present. In the trauma setting, the radiographic study of choice is the computed tomography or CT scan. It is rapid, can assess the eye and orbit in multiple planes, and does not affect ferromagnetic objects which may be present in trauma. Just as comparing both eyes clinically is important to determine if trauma is present, examining the CT and comparing the affected to the contralateral side is important. Eyeball shape and contour as well as location can point to significant trauma. Obviously, the eyeball in the CT sequence should be round in caliber; a distorted contour is highly suspicious for severe trauma and may be predictive of poor visual outcomes. A globe that is subluxed out of the orbit or sunken in the eye socket also may be a sign of significant ocular trauma.

The dislocation of the native intraocular lens either posteriorly or outside the eyeball also can be visualized.

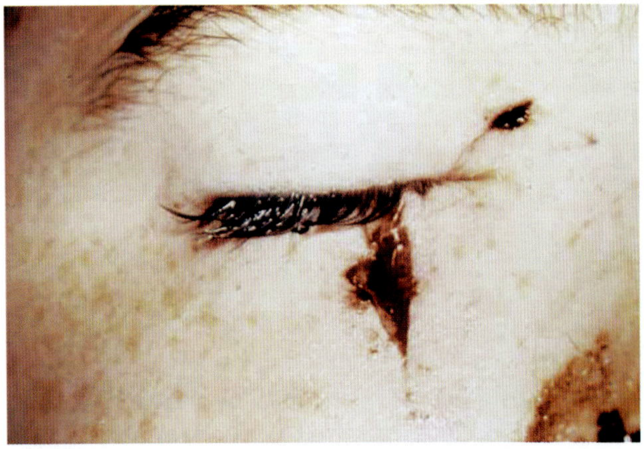

Fig 4–1. Full-thickness eyelid laceration is suspicious for a ruptured globe.

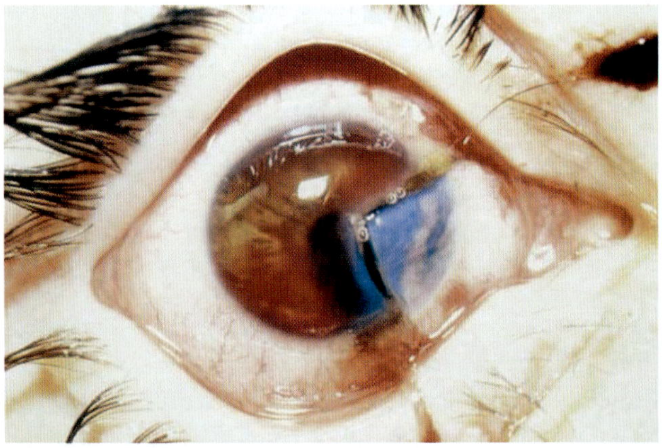

Fig 4–2. Careful elevation of lacerated eyelid reveals a corneal laceration.

Such trauma can be visualized with the presence of air or hemorrhage in the globe. Also foreign bodies, and in particular, ferromagnetic objects which appear hyperintense can be present in the eye socket or orbit. Often one can see a trail of air pointing to the presence of a foreign body in the eye or eye socket. The presence of any of these should raise suspicion for a ruptured globe. Finally, periocular fractures, of the nose or orbital bones, are telling of significant force being transmitted to the eye and possibly causing damage.

If a ruptured globe is suspected and the patient is otherwise medically stable, arrangements should be made for surgical exploration of the eyeball to find and repair all ruptures. Timing of such repairs should be within 24 hours to decrease the risk of associated infection and endophthalmitis. Until surgery, broad-spectrum intravenous antibiotics are indicated as well as shielding the eye to prevent further manipulation and damage to the globe. Finally, other periocular injuries and interventions to be repaired should be delayed until all intraocular issues are settled.

TRAUMATIC OPTIC NEUROPATHY

Traumatic optic neuropathy (TON) is damage to the optic nerve, and should be suspected when a patient has facial trauma with decreased vision but no obvious eye damage. Patients with TON complain of decreased vision. On examination, their vision can be variably depressed from minimal decrease of vision to complete loss of vision. Pupil examination often reveals abnormality on the swinging penlight test. Color vision is often affected as well as peripheral vision. An easy way to test color vision is to find a red object, and determine if a patient sees the intensity of the red color differently in each eye. An eye with optic nerve dysfunction will note that the red appears paler or pinkish in the affected side.

Although there are many classifications of TON describing the modality of injury, the most common cause is shearing or compression of nerve fibers at the level of the optic canal. This is due to the dural sheath's (of the optic nerve) firm attachment to the bone of the canal.

Treatment for TON is manifold and controversial. The treatment can include high-dose intravenous steroids and orbital canal decompression. Studies such as the International Optic Nerve Trauma Study in 1999[2] attempted to analyze the efficacy of steroids at the time of diagnosis but no definitive results were found in part due to the varied presentation of TON and that some patients had improvement of vision without intervention. Since then, some authors including Steinsapir[3] have commented that high-dose steroids may be detrimental to recovery. Likewise, optic canal decompression has been demonstrated by some to be effective, but in all studies, no controls were used to determine true efficacy of the intervention. This is exemplified by a recent report by Shibuya[4]; although this retrospective analysis tried to determine if fracture repair in the presence of TON caused decline in visual acuity, visual improvement was similar in groups that have fracture repair with steroid therapy (75%) or steroid therapy alone (64%). In those with optic nerve decompression, vision improvement was much lower (30%) and visual decline was seen (20%). However, there was no standardization of therapy or which patients received therapy, so the data are not very useful. In the setting of TON, if a true canal fracture with bone fragments compressing the nerve is present or a foreign body is impinging on the nerve, a canal decompression makes sense.

ORBITAL COMPARTMENT SYNDROME

The orbital compartment syndrome is when elevation of intraorbital pressure causes impairment of vascular perfusion to the optic nerve and globe.[5] The causes of this are diverse including retrobulbar hemorrhage, emphysema, inflammation, infections, and neoplasms. External signs of the compartment syndrome include ecchymosis with tense eyelids which are difficult to open, proptosis, increase resistance to retropulsion, and limitation of ocular motility (Fig 4–3). The visual acuity and color vision can be variably decreased and pupil reaction is often abnormal.

Elevation of orbital pressure is possible in part because of the anatomy of the orbit. The orbit is defined by the four bony orbital walls posteriorly and bound anteriorly by the orbital septum. The septum is a fibrous sheath firmly attached to the orbital rim for 360 degrees. It then lies within the confines of the eyelid and inserts into the tarsus, or skeleton of the eyelids. Although the eyelids can move in a vertical fashion, they are rigidly fixated in the horizontal plane by the medial and lateral canthal tendon. Therefore, if any space-occupying lesion infiltrates the orbit, particularly in an acute fashion, the orbital pressure

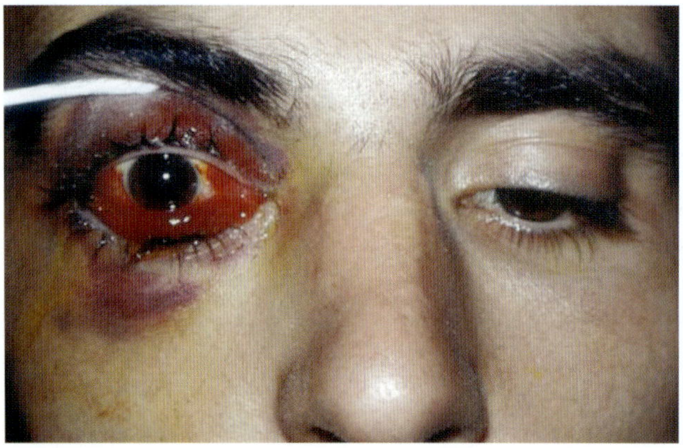

Fig 4–3. Elevation of tight eyelids reveal chemosis, proptosis, and limited motility.

will increase, often drastically. Blood infiltrating the orbital soft tissues can lead to a blinding retro-orbital hemorrhage, and a rapidly advancing orbital abscess can have a similar effect. Even iatrogenic increase of orbital pressure from surgical packing can cause vision loss.

As the orbit is bound by the septum and the canthal tendons, release of orbital pressure is best accomplished by release of the lateral canthal tendon via a lateral canthotomy and cantholysis (Figs 4–4, 4–5, and 4–6). The first step is the lateral canthotomy. Under local anesthesia, a horizontal incision through the lateral commisure and the lateral canthus is made with surgical scissors. The incision's length is approximately 6 mm extending to the orbital rim. The second and more important step is the inferior cantholysis. The lateral portion of the lower eyelid is grasped with toothed forceps and retracted away from the globe. Scissors are pointed toward the tip of the nose and used to palpate the now visible inferior crus of the lateral canthal tendon. The crus is then lysed allowing complete eversion and distraction of the lower eyelid away from the globe. Usually this incision is accompanied by forward luxation of the globe. This will not damage the optic nerve and actually allows decompression of the orbital pressure. Neither evacuation of the blood, nor removal of bone is necessary to decompress the orbit. Postsurgical management can include orbital imaging, and prophylactic antibiotics. Reattachment of the lateral canthal tendon is often not necessary, but if required can be pursued 1 to 2 weeks after initial intervention.

Orbital compartment syndrome is a true emergency because elevated orbital pressure for greater than 90 minutes can cause irreversible optic nerve damage. As such, the compartment syndrome is a clinical diagnosis and orbital imaging should not be pursued to confirm its presence. Therefore, any suspected orbital compartment syndrome should be reversed rapidly via canthotomy and cantholysis.

ORBITAL FRACTURE WITH MUSCLE ENTRAPMENT

One sequela of periocular trauma is an orbital fracture. These fractures can occur in isolation or in combination with other facial fractures and laceration(s). Most fractures can be evaluated and repaired in a timely fashion (usually 1–2 weeks after initial insult). However, one scenario exists in which urgent intervention is warranted—orbital fracture with muscle entrapment. This fracture pattern usually presents with a young patient (under 18 years of age) with blunt trauma to the periocular region. External signs can include a quiet, white eye with restriction of motility opposite the location of the fracture (Fig 4–7). This constellation of signs is often associated with nausea and vomiting and bradycardia—both part of the oculocardiac reflex. These findings are confirmed by many studies including one by Baek and Lee.[6] In this small series of 17 pediatric patients, 13 had muscle entrapment, 9 had nausea/vomiting (N/V), and 5 had bradycardia. All patients with N/V or bradycardia had resolution of symptoms after surgery.

Enophthalmos is not typical with diagnosis. On examination, decreased motility can be confirmed by forced ductions. Under topical anesthesia, toothed forceps are used to grasp medially and laterally to test vertical ductions. With the patient trying to look up, the eye is slowly

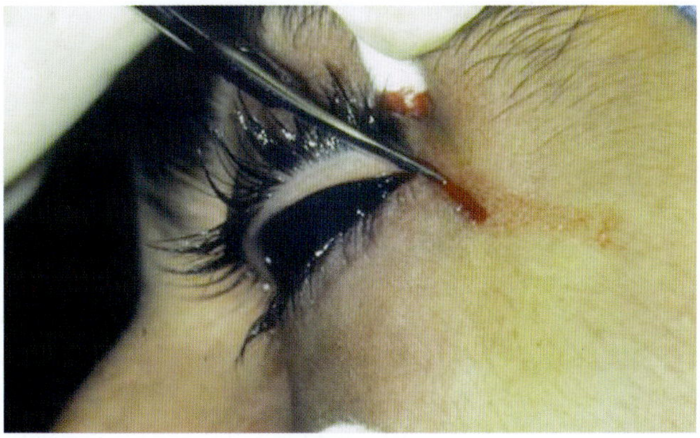

Fig 4–4. The horizontal incision through the lateral commisure and canthus is the first part of the lateral canthotomy/cantholysis.

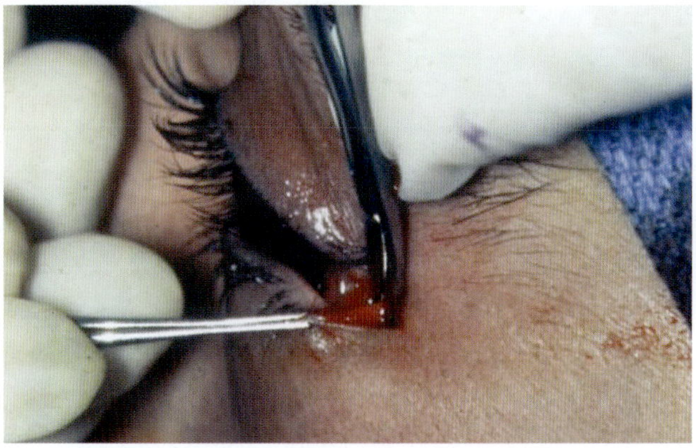

Fig 4–5. The eyelid is distracted away from the globe and inferior crus of the canthal tendon is palpated and bisected.

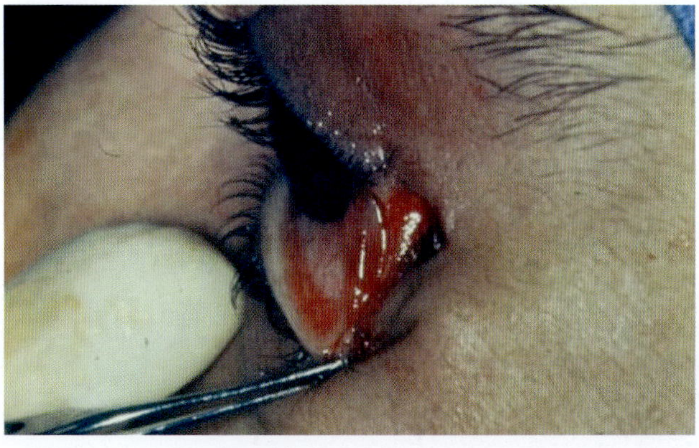

Fig 4–6. Complete release of the inferior crus allows complete distraction of the eyelid from the globe.

pulled in the same direction and presence of resistance is determined; if resistance to duction is encountered, then entrapped soft tissue into a fracture should be suspected. If restriction is not encountered, another etiology for decreased motility such as muscle paralysis should be entertained.

Imaging studies will help define the injury. CT scans of the orbit with coronal cuts will help visualize fractures with suspected entrapment. In such cases, a small fracture with adjacent soft tissue in or past the fracture plane is suggestive of entrapment (Fig 4–8). The key is that the imaging study is suggestive of entrapment; like the orbital compartment syndrome, fractures with entrapment are a clinical diagnosis. Another sign of possible entrapment is a change in shape of the rectus muscle next to a fracture. For example, the inferior rectus usually has a horizontal, elliptical shape on coronal images. Distortion of this shape, to a more vertical or round appearance, can suggest entrapment of soft tissues associated with muscle in an adjacent fracture.

This fracture pattern of entrapment is most common in the pediatric population, most likely due to the flexibility of the young orbital bones compared to the more brittle orbital bones in the adult. When blunt trauma occurs in the pediatric orbit, the flexible bone breaks linearly creating a trap door. This trap door opens and soft tissue is dragged into the defect. The trap door then closes entrapping the soft tissue. In the adult orbit, the bones typically shatter causing larger defects which do not entrap soft tissue. Instead these large defects cause enophthalmos. The most common wall affected by this fracture pattern is the orbital floor followed by the medial wall.

Intervention for fractures should be performed on an urgent basis, within 24 to 48 hours. If intervention is delayed, irreversible damage to the muscle can ensue, causing permanent double vision and ocular motility problems.

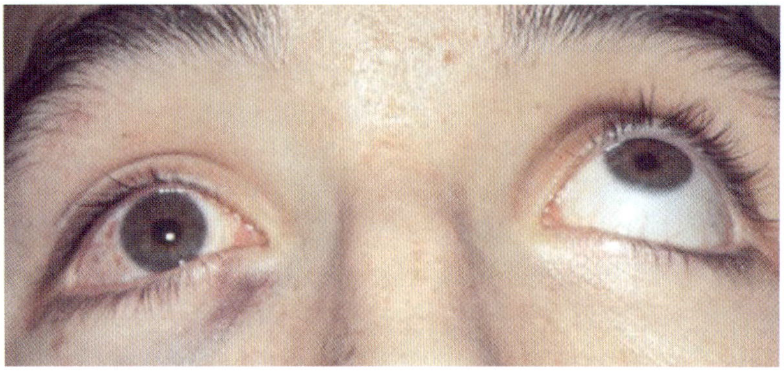

Fig 4–7. Limited motility of the right eye on up-gaze with a quiet eye is suggestive of orbital fracture with muscle entrapment.

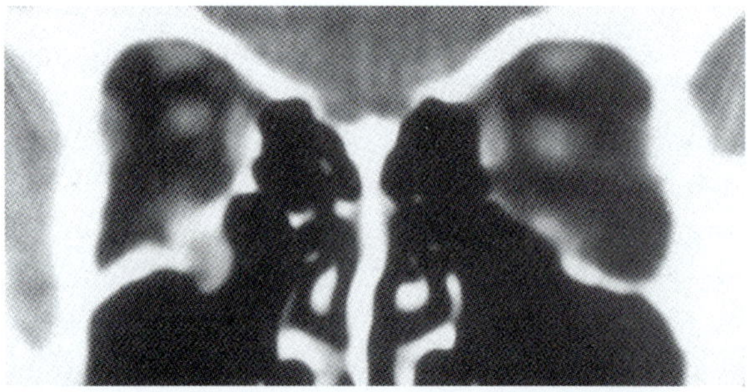

Fig 4–8. Coronal CT of the patient in Figure 4-7 reveals a small linear fracture of the orbital floor with soft tissue past the normal plane of the floor and helps confirm the diagnosis of orbital fracture with entrapment.

The goal of surgery should be the release of entrapped tissue and the closure of fractures. Although there are many approaches to the orbit for fracture repairs, a direct approach either transconjunctivally for orbital floor fractures or transcaruncularly for medial wall fractures is advised. Once the subperiosteal plane is established, the fracture should be visualized and an attempt should be made to release the soft tissue with blunt dissection and gentle traction. Often the fracture needs to be opened and enlarged to allow complete release of entrapped tissue. Once all entrapped tissue is released, the fracture is reduced and repaired by repositioning the fractured bones and plating with various materials. With these smaller fractures, often absorbable plates or even a sheet of gel film is adequate to allow the fracture to close without integration of the soft tissue into the scar. Forced ductions should be repeated throughout the procedure to confirm the reduction of the entrapment. Even after successful release of soft tissue, ocular motility may not approach normal function for weeks; however, forced ductions during this healing period, if repeated, should be negative.

CONCLUSION

In dealing with periocular trauma, most injuries can be repaired in a timely fashion. However, there are a few emergencies that require prompt clinical diagnosis and urgent treatment. These include ruptured globes, traumatic optic neuropathy, orbital compartment syndrome, and orbital fracture with muscle entrapment. Successful management of these emergencies will then allow the clinician to safely proceed with proper restoration of orbital and periocular anatomy.

Acknowledgment. All photographic images are courtesy of Peter A. D. Rubin, M.D.

REFERENCES

1. Chang EL, Bernardino CR, Watkins, LM, Rubin, PAD. Letter to the Editor: Rebleed of traumatic hyphema after closed reduction of nasal fracture. *J Cranio-Maxillofacial Surg.* 2003;31:191–192.
2. Levin LA, Beck RW, Joseph MP, et al. The treatment of traumatic optic neuropathy: the international optic nerve trauma study. *Ophthalmology.* 1999;106:1268–1277.
3. Steinsapir KD. Treatment of traumatic optic nerve with high-dose corticosteroid. *J Neuro-Ophthalmol.* 2006;26:65–67.
4. Shibuya TY, Feinberg SM, Mathog RH L, et al. Visual risks of facial fracture repair in the setting of traumatic optic neuropathy. *Arch Otolaryngol Head Neck Surg.* 2006;132:258–264.
5. Linberg JV. Orbital compartment syndromes following trauma. *Adv Ophthalmic Plast Reconstr Surg.* 1987;6:51–62.
6. Baek SH, Lee EY. Clinical analysis of internal orbital fractures in children. *Korean J Ophthalmol.* 2003;17(1):44–49.

5

Pediatric Mandibular Fractures

Steven Roser

The incidence of facial fractures in children is significantly less than adults.[1] Mandible fractures make up a higher percentage of facial fractures in children. Falls from bicycles, skateboards, stairs, or almost any other raised object are responsible for the majority of isolated mandibular fractures.[2] All types of sports can result in mandible fractures in children. In sports, usually it is contact between two children, such as face to knee, that results in fracture. Automobiles and other motorized vehicular accidents result in mandibular fractures, but usually these children have other injuries, including head, chest, abdominal, and extremity injuries, many of which are significant. Maxillofacial surgeons on call at hospitals that are designated Level II trauma centers and below will most commonly be caring for the isolated pediatric facial fractures. The high-impact injuries will be cared for by those on staff at the Level I trauma centers. Although child abuse infrequently results in facial fractures,[3] the possibility must be ruled out.

Although the soft and hard tissue anatomy is basically similar in the adult and the child, the differences provide significant challenges to the treatment of mandibular fractures in the child. From birth until age 12 years, the child will have developing teeth within the jaws. The deciduous teeth are developing within the mandible at birth. By age 2, most children will have erupted these teeth and the permanent tooth buds will be present. The developing tooth buds occupy the entire mandible leaving no room for the placement of screws for fixation plates (Fig 5–1). From 2 to 4 years old, the deciduous teeth roots have not been resorbed enough to loosen or result in exfoliation and the teeth can be used to support a variety of wiring techniques. However, the crowns of the posterior deciduous teeth are bell shaped and make it difficult to wire on an arch bar.

From age 4 years and older, starting with the incisors, the child begins to exfoliate the deciduous dentition and erupt the permanent dentition. During the next 6 years the patient is in a mixed dentition stage, that is, a combination of exfoliating deciduous teeth and erupting permanent teeth which may result in too few teeth to place wires for maxillomandibular fixation.

The mandible is usually the last bone in the body to complete growth.[4] The impact of the injury and the fracture repair on the growing mandible must be taken into account when planning treatment. Mandibular growth is in a downward and forward direction as a result of the forces placed on it by the muscle and ligamentous attachments. The condyle has been traditionally considered as a growth center under both hormonal and muscle/ligament influence. Injury to the condyle and subsequent immobility can result in ankylosis and significant restriction of growth. The posterior border of the ramus and the alveolar ridge are other areas of the mandible in which growth occurs. The application of titanium plates on the growing mandible carries the risk of growth restriction. This plus the potential damage done by screws to the developing toothbuds must be kept in mind when considering using plates for fracture stabilization. In addition to growth potential, other considerations that must be taken into account in the treatment of mandible fractures in children are rapid healing and varying degrees of cooperation.

DIAGNOSIS

In adults, approximately 60% of mandible fractures involve the angle and the subcondylar region. In children, fractures of this area account for 80% of all mandibular factures. Symphysis and parasymphysis fractures are more common in children than adults.[5]

The diagnosis of mandibular fractures in children, similar to adults, starts with a history. It is more common for the fractures of the mandible in children to correlate with the severity of the impact. Usually there are abrasions or lacerations present which can help alert the examiner to potential bony trauma (Fig 5–2). Most children who are able to speak can tell the examiner where it hurts. In adults, the presence of a recognizable malocclusion often accompanies a mandibular fracture. In children the mixed dentition can obscure a malocclusion that is the result of a fracture. However, the finding of an open bite, anterior or unilateral posterior, should make one suspicious of the presence of fractures especially subcondylar factures which are common in children. Other important signs of subcondylar fractures in children include lack of opening or deviation on opening to the side of the injury. Because the presence of a malocclusion is key to both making the diagnosis and the treatment, the examiner should determine this before palpating the area of injury which usually causes pain and can result in the child refusing to cooperate further with being examined. Also prior to palpation, the examiner should look at the floor of the mouth for a sublingual hematoma which is seen almost 100% of the time with a symphyseal fracture.

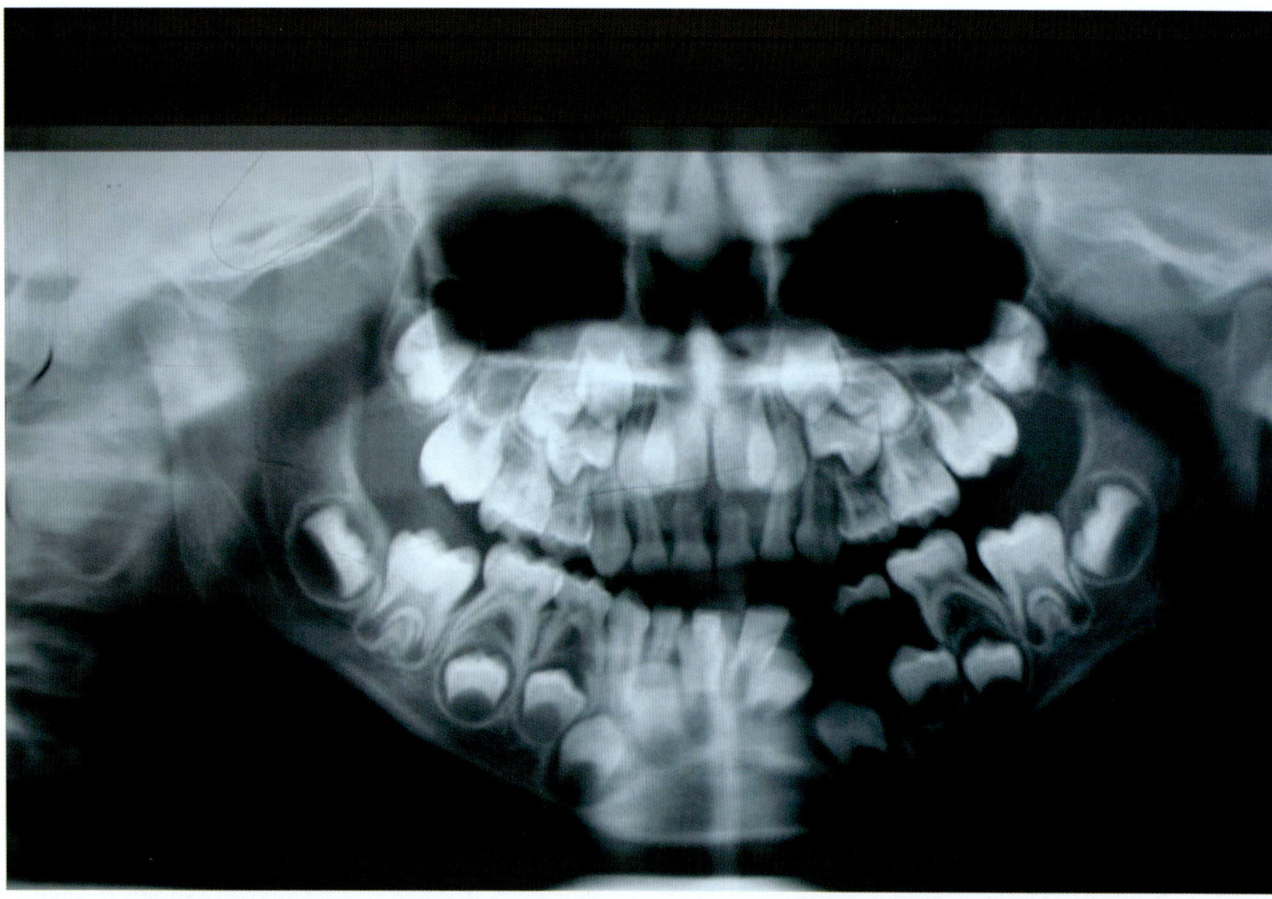

Fig 5–1. Panoramic radiograph of a 3½-year-old patient. Note presence of developing tooth buds of permanent dentition near the inferior border of the mandible.

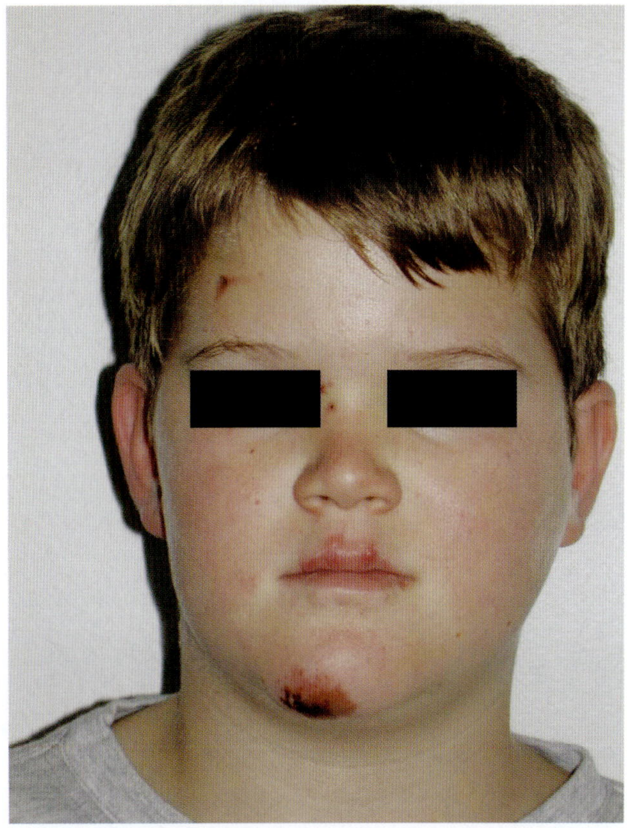

Fig 5–2. Seven-year-old patient with a fracture of the left condyle resulting from a fall. Note the abrasion on the chin.

Fractures in the symphyseal and parasymphyseal region are often greenstick or only minimally displaced in the child and can be difficult to see on plain films. Like adults with mandibular trauma, children will have two fractures more often than one making it important to search for the second. The combinations of fractures are similar in the child as the adult with the symphysis/parasymphysis being accompanied by a condylar fracture on the contralateral side. Radiographs become more important in diagnosing mandible fractures in children because of the lack of cooperation which may limit the exam. Almost all children who present with mandibular fractures are seen in the emergency room as opposed to adults who often are referred to surgeon's offices. In children as well as adults, the panoramic radiograph is a useful plain film (Fig 5–3). The panoramic film needs to be accompanied by a second view such as a PA mandible, Towne's view, or an occlusal radiograph. Lack of cooperation particularly in an injured young child will preclude these views and the CT scan, particularly the spiral CT, takes only a few minutes and often does not require sedation. In Level I and II trauma centers, CT scans are routinely obtained on children with facial trauma (Figs 5–4 and 5–5). Displacement of mandibular fractures, particularly subcondylar, are well seen on reformatted 3-dimensional CT scans. The presence and severity of the malocclusion and the amount of pain the child is experiencing from the fracture are important elements forming the basis of the management plan.

TREATMENT

Although the basic principles of fracture repair are the same for children as adults, the child presents some differences that will significantly alter the treatment planning.

The healing of a bone fracture in children begins almost immediately and is well underway in days.[6] Therefore, it is necessary to make the diagnosis and implement the treatment quickly. In adults fracture healing allows for

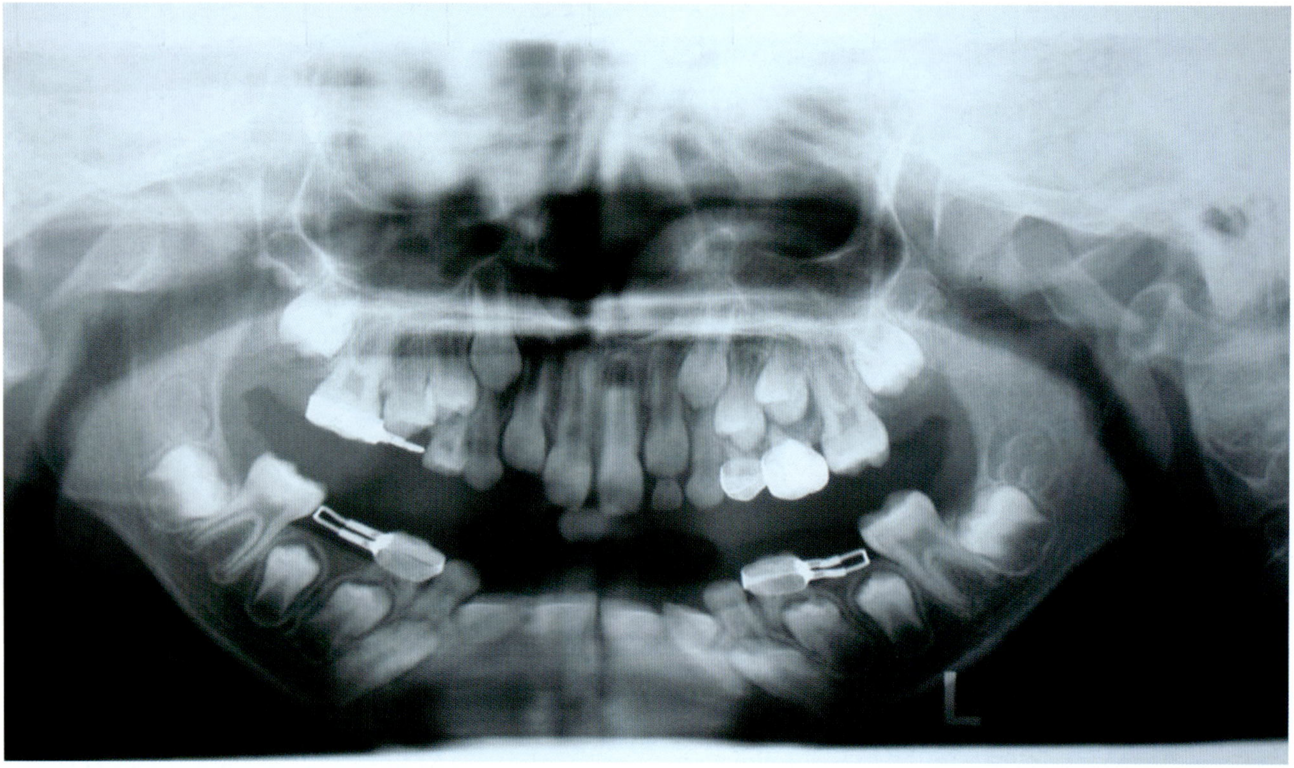

Fig 5–3. Panoramic radiograph of a 6-year-old patient in a mixed dentition.

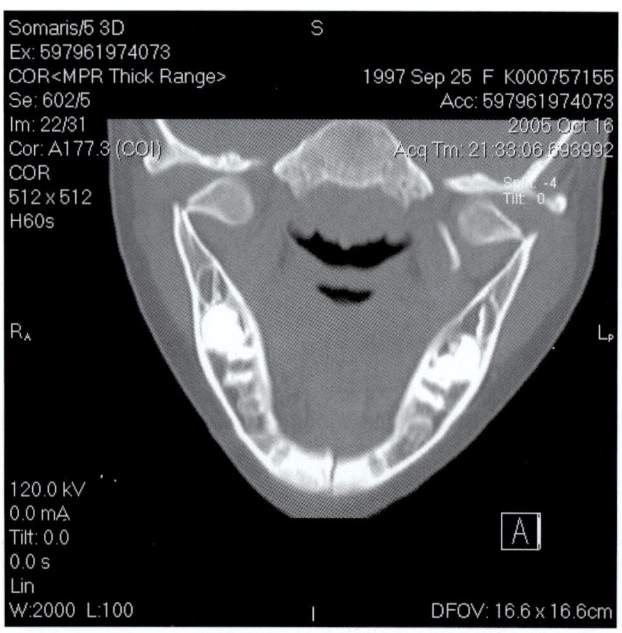

Fig 5–4. CT scan illustrating bilateral condylar fractures with anteromedial displacement of proximal segments.

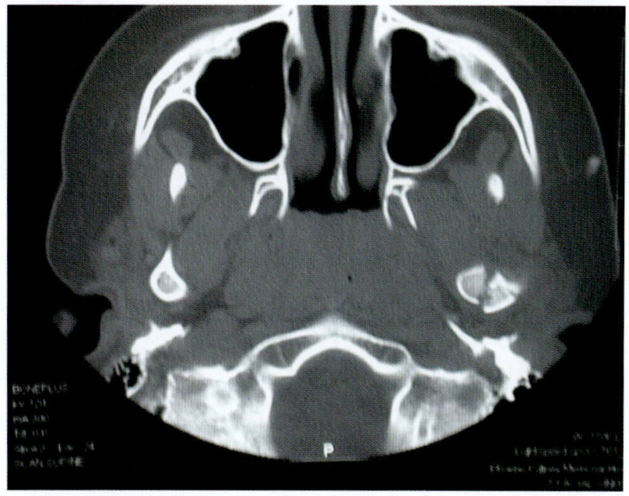

Fig 5–5. CT scan illustrating intra-articular fracture of the left condyle.

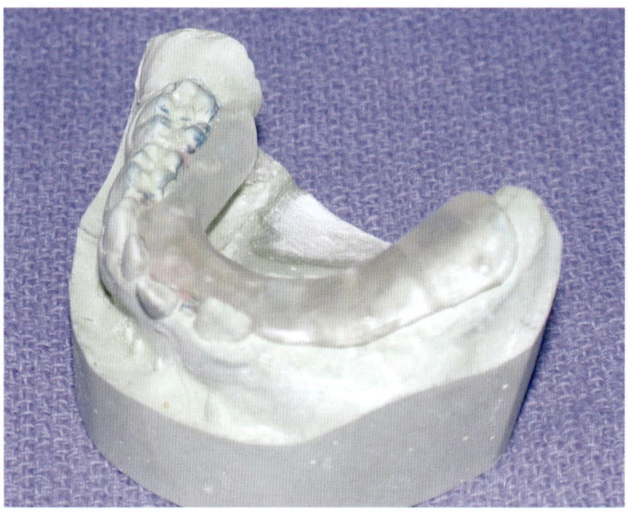

Fig 5–6. Acrylic splint constructed to stabilize symphysis fracture in a 5-year-old. This splint will be fixed with a combination of wires around the deciduous teeth on the right side and circumandibular wires on the parasymphysis and left body area.

a window of up to 14 days before closed manipulation of the fracture becomes impossible. In children this window can be as short as 7 days. The developing dentition presents differences that will alter treatment. The presence of the developing tooth buds in the child under 10 may preclude the use of plate fixation. The mixed dentition with many missing deciduous teeth and not fully erupted permanent teeth, may preclude the use of arch bars or other interdental techniques used for maxillomandibular fixation. Lastly, the lack of understanding of the injury and need for treatment by the young child may lead to significant lack of cooperation and may preclude the use of maxillomandibular fixation.

FRACTURES OF THE SYMPHYSIS AND BODY

Most of these fractures are greenstick, undisplaced, or minimally displaced. This is the result of the more elastic nature of the mandible in the child or the presence of the toothbuds which can hold the mandible together. If the only fracture is in this area, a soft diet may be all that is necessary for healing and the erupting teeth will make up small occlusal discrepancies that result from minimal displacement. If a significant step deformity exists, closed management with a 2-week period of maxillomandibular fixation (MMF) may be required. If the child lacks the dentition to wire together, a number of alternatives are available. The first is a lingual splint. This is a custom-made acrylic splint that is wired to the available teeth in the mandibular arch or secured with circumandibular wires (Fig 5–6). The device is made from a set of models which may need to be obtained under general anesthesia. The mandibular model is cut at the fracture sites and the segments reduced and glued together. The placement of the lingual splint usually requires a second general anesthetic. Usually the child does not need to be placed in MMF and can eat soft foods. The splint can be removed in 3 weeks and usually requires a general anesthetic for removal. Maxillomandibular fixation can be achieved without interdental wiring by using circumandibular wires, circumzygomatic wires, and piriform rim wires. These can be painful and require a general anesthetic for removal. Each child presents their own set of challenges and the treating surgeon should be prepared to think creatively regarding the design of custom devices, interdental wiring, and circumskeletal and intraosseous fixation. In the 6 to 12-year-old child there may be enough room to place a 2.0-mm titanium plate at the inferior border using monocortical screws. This system is load sharing and requires at least consideration of additional stabilization methods like MMF or dietary restrictions. Developing toothbuds both permanent and deciduous are resilient and usually survive fractures running through the area where they are located. The surgeon should alert the parents to the possibility of the failure of the toothbud/s to further develop or that ankylosis of the developing tooth may occur. This needs to be monitored over time and information about the fracture and the treatment should be transmitted to the child's pediatric dental provider.

ANGLE FRACTURES

Angle fractures in children occur far less commonly than in adults. Because the child does not have an impacted third molar to serve as an area of weakness, the forces are transmitted to the conylar area and the fractures occur there. Nondisplaced fractures whether favorable or unfavorable are treated by closed management. If the family and child seem cooperative, a soft diet for 3 weeks may be adequate. If cooperation is not forthcoming, 3 weeks of MMF may be required. Displaced mobile fractures may require an open reduction. There may be enough room to place a small plate to stabilize the segments and MMF may still be required. Wire osteosynthesis should be considered as it will permit stabilization and is less invasive than plates and screws. In older children, there may be room to place 2.0 miniplates fixed with monocortical screws. As mentioned above this is a load-sharing system and may require additional stabilization methods. Resorbable plates are not being used currently for the repair of mandibular fractures. Continuing progress in the size, strength, and resorption time of resorbable plates will undoubtly make these plates the device of choice for fracture repair in the child. Similar to symphysis and body fractures, angle fractures that are displaced, but not grossly, can be allowed to heal in that position. Normal function and growth will make up for small bone/occlusal discrepancies.

CONDYLAR FRACTURES

The treatment of condylar fractues in the child remains controversial, perhaps less so than the adult. Because falls are the most common etiology of mandible fractures in the child, trauma to the chin usually occurs. The forces are routinely transmitted to the condyles resulting in injury to the condyle and temporomandibular joint. These injuries include hemarthrosis, intracapsular fractures, simple and comminuted, and nondisplaced and displaced subcondylar fractures. Because the condylar neck in the child is short and thus less likely to break, the forces are more commonly transmitted to the condyle and intracapsular fractures are more common in the child. A typical fracture is a vertical split of the condyle with medial displacement of the medial pole (see Fig 5–5). Condylar fractures in children are classified in a similar manner as adults such as unilateral or bilateral, displaced or dislocated out of the fossa.[7] In children, however, the type of fracture is not as important in the treatment planning as the pain on function the child is experiencing, the child's age, the presence of a mixed dentition, and perhaps most importantly the presence of an open bite malocclusion. Open reduction of the condyle is rarely indicated in the young child. The only exception would be if the displaced fracture segments are mechanically interfering with function.[1,5,8]

If the child can function without significant pain and does not have a significant malocclusion, observation and a soft diet for 1 to 2 weeks usually is adequate. If the child has considerable pain and or a significant open bite malocclusion, 2 weeks of MMF should be considered. If the lack of teeth or other conditions make the prospect of MMF particularly challenging, in children with unilateral condylar fractures, analgesics, liquid diet, and observation for a few days is indicated. Decreased pain and muscle spasm may allow the restoration of enough function and reduction or elimination of the malocclusion thus eliminating the need for intervention. After 1 to 2 weeks and the resolution of pain, if the child is old enough to follow direction, jaw opening and stretching exercises should be prescribed. Open bite malocclusions as the result of displaced bilateral condylar fractures usually requires a period of MMF. In the older child with persistence of the open bite malocclusion after 2 weeks of MMF, restoration of shortened ramus height using an open reduction either directly or endoscopically should be considered.[9,10] Prolonged immobility, beyond 2 to 3 weeks, can result in hypomobility. Children under 3 years of age are particularly vulnerable to condylar fractures producing bony ankylosis.[1] Significant hypomobility either as the result of fibrous or bony ankylosis with limited function will result in significant growth restriction of the affected side (Fig 5–7). In younger children with condylar fractures without limited function, remodeling often occurs with restoration of normal function and no interference with mandibular growth.[11] Most observers report the younger the child the more likely the remodeling to normal condylar morphology is to occur. However, even with lack of remodeling most children continued to grow normally and had no restriction of function.[11,12]

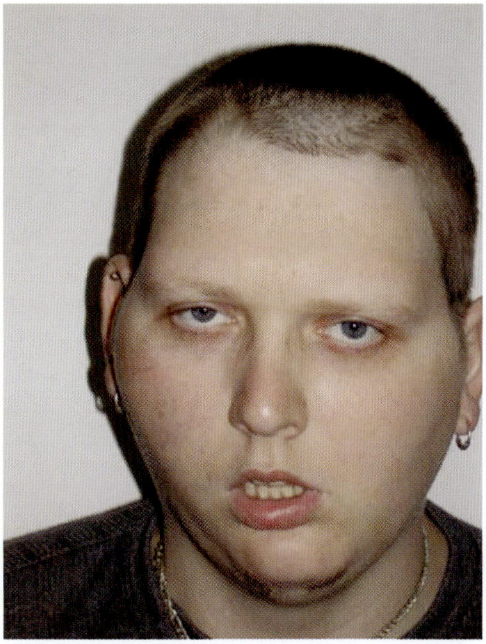

Fig 5–7. Fracture of the left condyle at age 8 years has resulted in asymmetric mandibular growth in this 20-year-old.

REFERENCES

1. Dodson TB. Mandibular fractures in children. *OMS Knowledge Update.*1995; 1(pt II):95–107.
2. Iida S, Matsuya T. Pediatric maxillofacaial fractures; their aetiological characters and fracture patterns. *J Craniomaxillofac Surg.* 2002;30:237–241.
3. Needleman HI. Orofacial trauma in child abuse: types, prevalence, management and the dental profession's involvement. *Pediatr Dent.* 1986;8:71–80.
4. Kaban LB. Facial trauma. II. Dentoalveolar injuries and mandibular fractures. In: Kaban LB, ed. *Pediatric Oral and Maxillofacial Surgery.* Philadelphia, Pa: WB Saunders; 2004:446.
5. Kaban LB, Mullikan JB, Murray JE. Facial fractures in children, an analysis of 122 fractures in 109 patients. *Plast Reconst Surg.* 1977;59:15–20.
6. Schultz RC, Meilman J. Facial fractures in children. In: Goldwyn RM, ed. *Long-Term Results in Plastic and Reconstructive Surgery.* Boston, Mass: Little Brown; 1980; 458–480.
7. Sorel B. Mandibular condylar fractures. *OMS Knowledge Update.* 2001;3:47–62.
8. Leake DJ, Doykos J, Habal HB. Long-term follow-up of fractures of the mandibular condyle in children. *J Plast Reconstruct Surg.* 1971;47:127–131.
9. Stobl H, Emhoff R, Rothler G. Conservative treatment of unilateral condylar fractures in children: a long-term clinical and radiological follow-up of 55 patients, *Int J Oral Maxillofac Surg* 1999;28:95–98.
10. Lee C, Mueller RV, Lee K, Mathes SJ. Endoscopic subcondylar fracture repair: functional esthetic and radiographic outcomes. *J Plas Reconstr Surg.* 1998;102:1434–1443.
11. Lund K. Mandibular growth and remodeling processes after condylar fracture: a longitudinal roentgencephalometric study. *Acta Odont Scand.* 1974; 32(suppl):3–117.
12. Norholt SE, Krishnan V, Sindet-Pedersen S, Jensen I. Pediatric condylar fractures: a long-term follow-up of 55 patients. *J Oral Maxillofac Surg.* 1993;51:1302–1310.

6

TRAUMA TO THE DEVELOPING TEETH

Michael P. Healey

Facial trauma in children often results in trauma to the teeth and supporting structures. Treatment of these incidents often varies between the age of the child, and the developmental stage of the face, head, and neck. Treatment decisions not only include the morphology and vitality of the tooth itself, but also how the incident may influence the formation and eruption of the permanent dentition. In addition, the role of the teeth in speech development, self-esteem, and the function of swallowing must be paramount in the practitioner's thought process. This chapter is designed to aid in a systematic plan that will restore the injured area and give the best long-term results.[1-4]

TRAUMA TO THE PRIMARY DENTITION: AGES 1 TO 5 YEARS

Trauma to the anterior primary teeth is very common in children. The very first concern should be that this child has suffered a head trauma and the first attention should be to rule out concussion and neurologic damage. When a parent calls after office hours, the doctor should insist on meeting the family at a facility where the appropriate help is present, such as a hospital emergency room. It is foolhardy to meet the family at a private office after hours, where in the event of a seizure, or worse, no help is immediately available. The initial oral examination includes an inspection of the injured area. If the tooth is in the same position as it was prior to the injury, palpate both the facial and lingual aspects of the alveolar bone supporting the teeth. Gently check for facial and lingual mobility. If the tooth or multiple teeth are mobile, assess the longevity of this area without stabilization (Figs 6–1 and 6–2). We rarely splint primary teeth because the child will most likely pick at the splint, and the periosteum will generally support the structure and will heal within 3 weeks. If the teeth will not hold their position, they will most likely require extraction. Next, gently retract the lips to check for intraoral lacerations. Labial frenums are extremely vascular and a small laceration can bleed profusely. Large lacerations may require suturing with 4-0 Vicryl. Check for vestibular lacerations. Lacerations in excess of 5 mm may require suturing. Oral mucosa in children is very friable and it can seem like you are suturing butter. Do not place much tension on these sutures. Finally, check to see if the child can bite the back teeth together. Inability to have a symmetric closure may be indicative of a mandibular or maxillary fracture. The mouth is a dirty area, and it is prudent to cover the child with amoxicillin or other appropriate antibiotic for 5 days after the injury if bleeding occurs.

SUBLUXATED TOOTH

When primary teeth are out of position, radiographs of the area are indicated prior to repositioning the teeth. These films will show if the root is fractured, or if the root of the tooth was prematurely resorbed from a prior injury. These teeth may not respond well to repositioning and may require extraction. Two views may be taken with a dental x-ray machine. The first is a periapical view. This either may be taken with the child holding the film with their lips, or the assistant holding the film with a pair of hemostats. Appropriate shielding should be observed. The second is an extraoral view with a size 00 film. This will show the

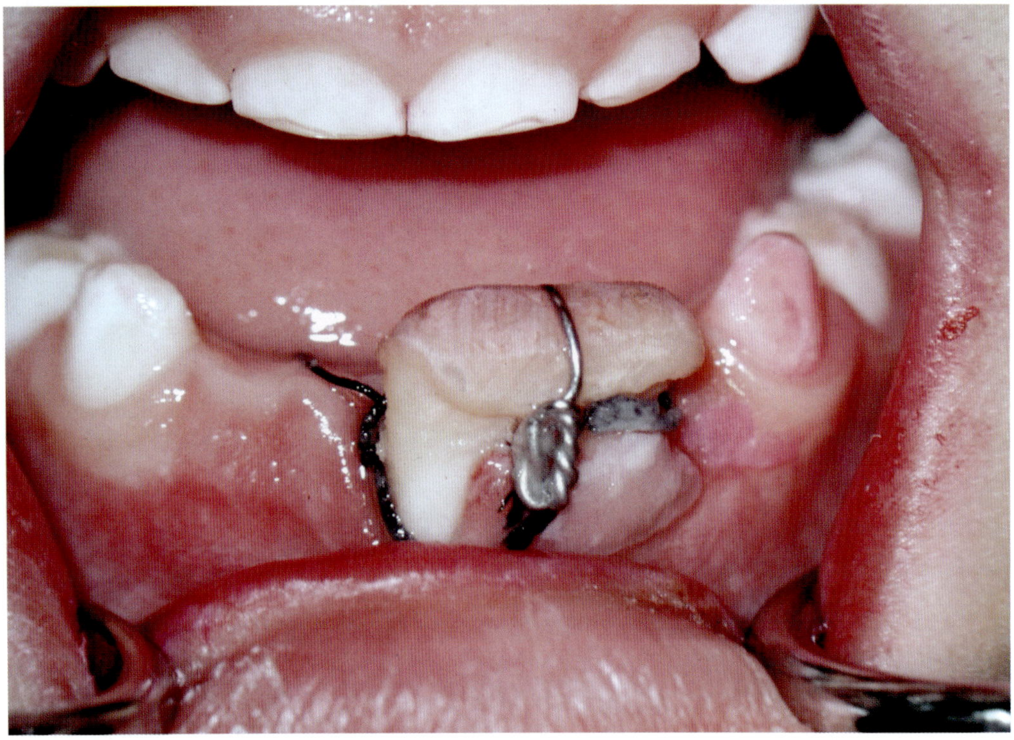

Fig 6–1. Stabilization of lower incisors with a splint and circumferential wire under the mandible.

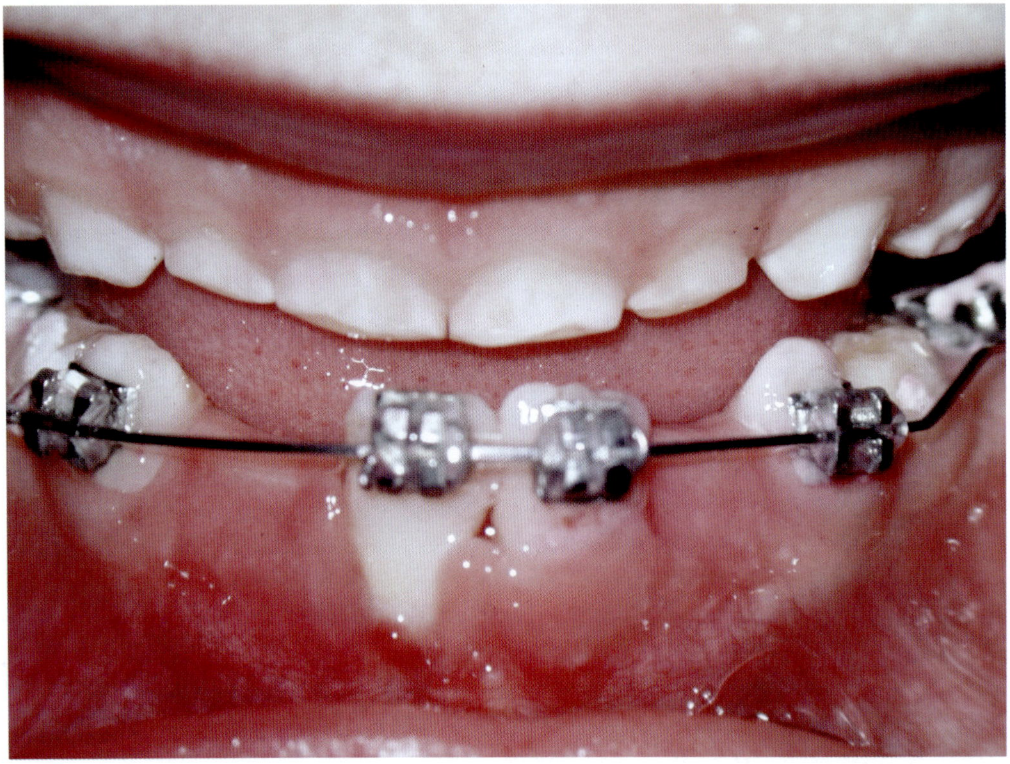

Fig 6–2. Photo demonstrating braces which are placed one week poststabilization of lower incisors (Fig 6–1).

position of the tooth in relation to the developing structures (Fig 6–3). When repositioning, the area requires a local anesthetic and a downward force to be applied, extruding the affected teeth to properly angle the tooth and the tooth reinserted to its proper position. If the crown is displaced to the lingual side, and one tries to just tip it

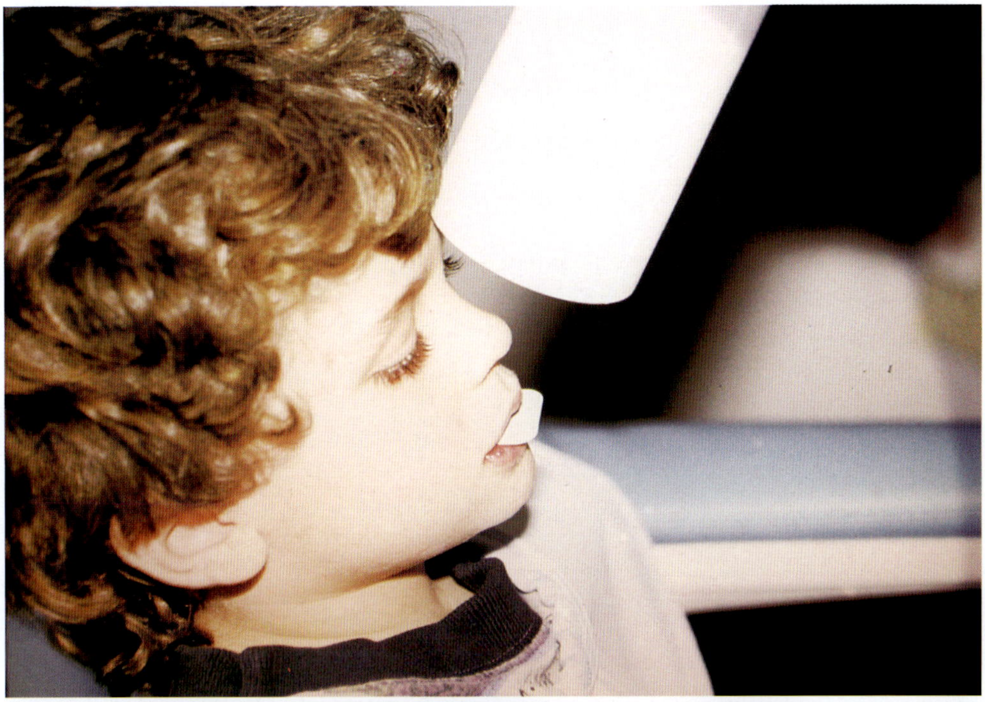

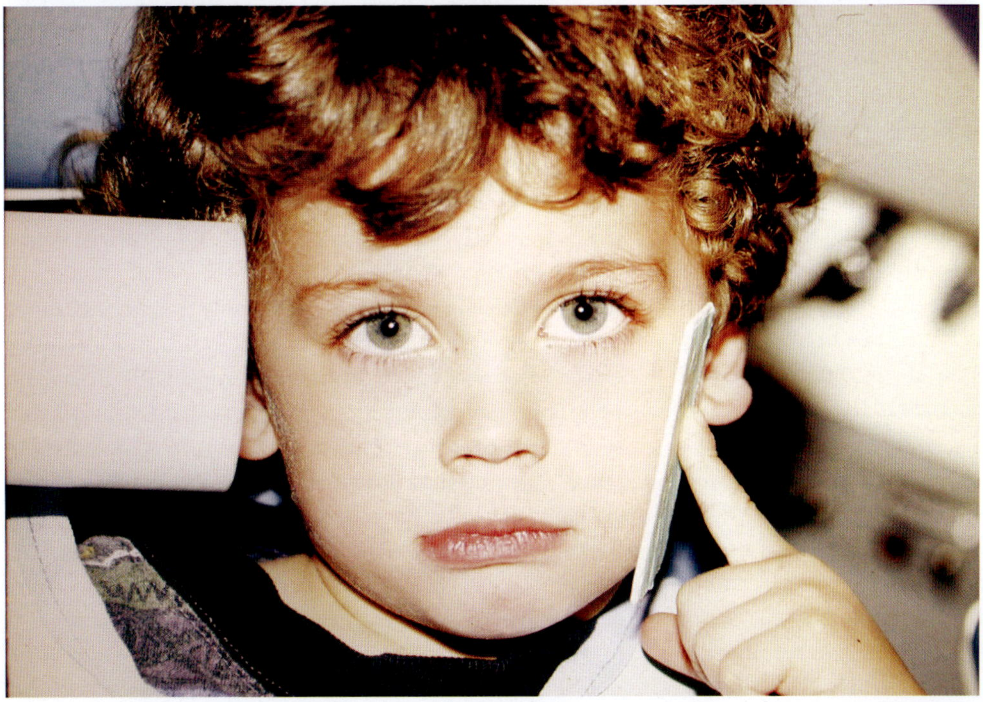

Fig 6–3A, B. Positioning of x-ray to determine tooth position.

forward, you risk breaking the root of the tooth. Check to see if the maxillary anterior tooth is in a facial position to the mandibular anterior teeth when the patient closes the teeth together for proper positioning. If the tooth remains essentially in the correct position within 2 to 3 mm, it will most likely heal. If the tooth will not retain its position, then it is better to extract it. Remember, we do not want to do anything that will do more damage to the developing permanent teeth that are still forming. Primary teeth may be repositioned up to 24 hours after the injury. If it has been longer than that, then one should not attempt to reposition it, and can wait to see if the lips will reposition the teeth over the first month.

If the tooth is invusled up to 4 mm, and the crown is visible, no treatment is necessary. The majority will re-erupt within 6 weeks. If it does not return to an acceptable position, then the tooth should be extracted. If the tooth is completely avulsed, then no matter how short a period of time, or what the storage medium it should *NOT* be reimplanted. Damage to the developing crown of the permanent tooth is common with heroically reimplanting avulsed deciduous teeth. Antibiotic coverage is indicated in all these injuries.[5]

TOOTH DISCOLORS AFTER INJURY

The pulp tissue of each primary tooth contains smooth muscle, unmylenated nerve fibers, and a vascular system, giving it a red coloration. Upon injury, the blood vessels can rupture creating bleeding into the dentin of the tooth, which is porous and has a very high organic component when compared to the enamel, and bleeding into the dentin will give a darkening of the tooth, often with no other apparent damage to the tooth. If the pulp tissue remains vital, the cellular activity will clean up the discolored dentin and the tooth will whiten (Fig 6–4). Often during the healing process, the cells will lay down reparative dentin and the pulp chamber will become radiographically obliterated. These teeth are healthy, and although they differ slightly in color from the adjacent teeth, most will exfoliate without problem and require no treatment.

If the pulp tissue loses its vitality, a different scenario occurs. Often an acute inflammatory reaction occurs in the pulp, increasing the hydrostatic pressure. As the dentin does not expand, the internal pressure inside the pulp can be higher than the blood pressure feeding it, so the part farthest away from the apex of the tooth can necrose. There is great variability as to the resiliency to the pulp tissue. This author has seen primary teeth that were grossly subluxated heal without incident, and the adjacent tooth necrose. Subsequent trauma can affect this healing process. It still takes 6 to 9 months for a damaged pulp to affect the surrounding structures. There are no bacteria involved in this process, so lengthy observation (3–5 months) prior to diagnosing the appropriate course of treatment is acceptable. If the color does not lighten and/or the tooth does not tighten, then irreversible pulpal damage has probably occurred. A pulpectomy, removing all the pulpal tissue and using a zinc-oxide and eugenol fill will generally stop any further damage. The color of the tooth can be restored with a composite crown. This author has found that once the area has been anesthetized, this pulpectomy can be completed in less than 10 minutes by using a No. 3 Gates Glidden bur on a low-speed handpiece, and injecting the zinc-oxide and eugenol paste with a centrix syringe. The fill should be at least 2 mm shy of the radiographic apex of the tooth. The newer bleaching shades of composite give a better result with the primary crown form than the A–1 shading. Once external root resorption occurs, the tooth must be extracted. A periapical cyst can alter the color and the shape of the permanent tooth. Of course, the length of time the tooth must remain, the behavior of the child, and the medical history must all be taken into consideration when deciding the appropriate course of treatment for a child.

FRACTURED PRIMARY TOOTH

Fractured teeth are classified by their location and the extent to which the tooth is involved. Fractures involving the enamel only are designated Ellis class I. A bright dental curing light can illuminate many of these that are not visible to the naked eye. These are the only fractures that may be restored by just recontouring the tooth, but extensive enamel fractures may require restoration with a composite filling material. Fractures involving the dentin (second layer of the tooth) are Ellis class II fractures. These require dental restoration. Some may be temporarily restored by trying to glue the fractured chip using the dentin bonding systems; however, these rarely last over 5 years. The deeper the vertical overbite, the greater will be the forces generated on the injured area and the poorer the prognosis for this repair. Restoration of fractures of this nature need not be restored immediately. In fact, a temporary sealant

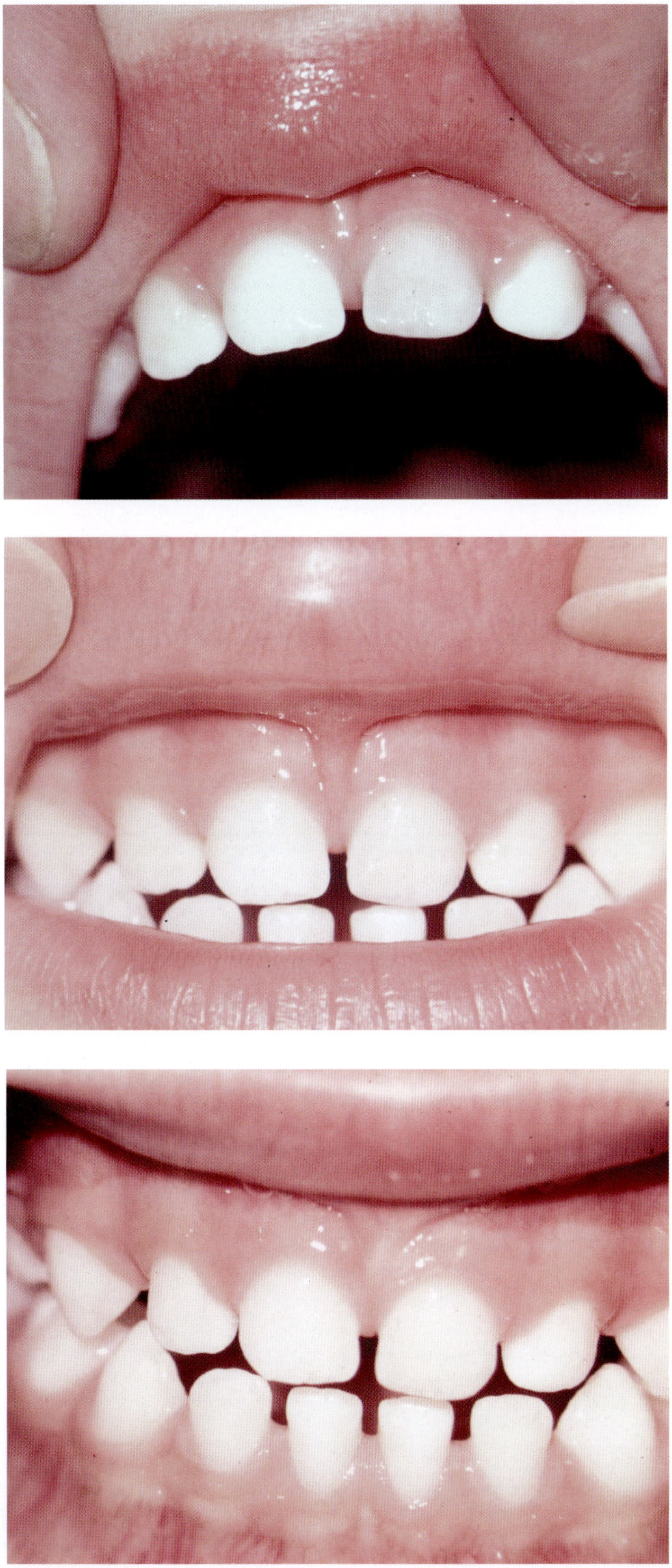

Fig 6–4A, B, C. Stepwise progression of primary tooth lightening with reparative dentition.

such as a glass ionomer (Fig 6–5) cement can allow time for the internal swelling of the pulpal tissues to subside, thereby increasing the probability that pulpal necrosis and endodontic treatment can be avoided. Fractures involving the pulpal tissue are Ellis class III and require treatment. Primary teeth that are fractured in this manner require endodontic treatment. Apical fill treatment has a more successful prognosis than a vital pulpotomy for anterior teeth. Vertical and horizontal root fractures in primary teeth require extraction of the tooth.

AVULSION OF PRIMARY TOOTH

Primary teeth that are avulsed are not reimplanted. The healing process often damages the formation of the permanent incisor teeth resulting in malformed crowns and defective enamel. It is safer to leave these teeth out and replace them with a fixed prosthetic appliance. Very small root fragments may be left and will be resorbed when the permanent tooth erupts; however, root tips and entire roots may damage the developing permanent incisor teeth when a chronic inflammatory reaction ensues (Fig 6–6).

REPLACEMENT OF MISSING ANTERIOR PRIMARY TEETH

Primary teeth are replaced with a prosthetic appliance known as a pediatric partial denture, or "pedo-partial" (Fig 6–7). Unlike a replacement for a permanent tooth, the adjacent teeth are not used for the anchorage points for these appliances. The abutment teeth are either the primary second molar, or the primary first molar teeth. The choice of restoration that anchors the prosthetic teeth are either an orthodontic band (Figs 6–8, 6–9, and 6–10) fitted around the primary second molars, or stainless steel crowns fitted to either the primary second molar, or the primary first molar teeth. The choice of abutment depends on the occlusion of the patient, and the restorative needs of the posterior teeth. The advantage of crowns on the primary first molar teeth is that the appliance has a shorter length of wire, flexes less, is more resistant to being dislodged than orthodontic bands, and forces the parent to seek care on at least an annual basis. When growth and development occur, the anterior portion of the maxillae grows downward faster than the posterior segment, so the prosthetic teeth appear to be pushed up into the gum tissue and are not in

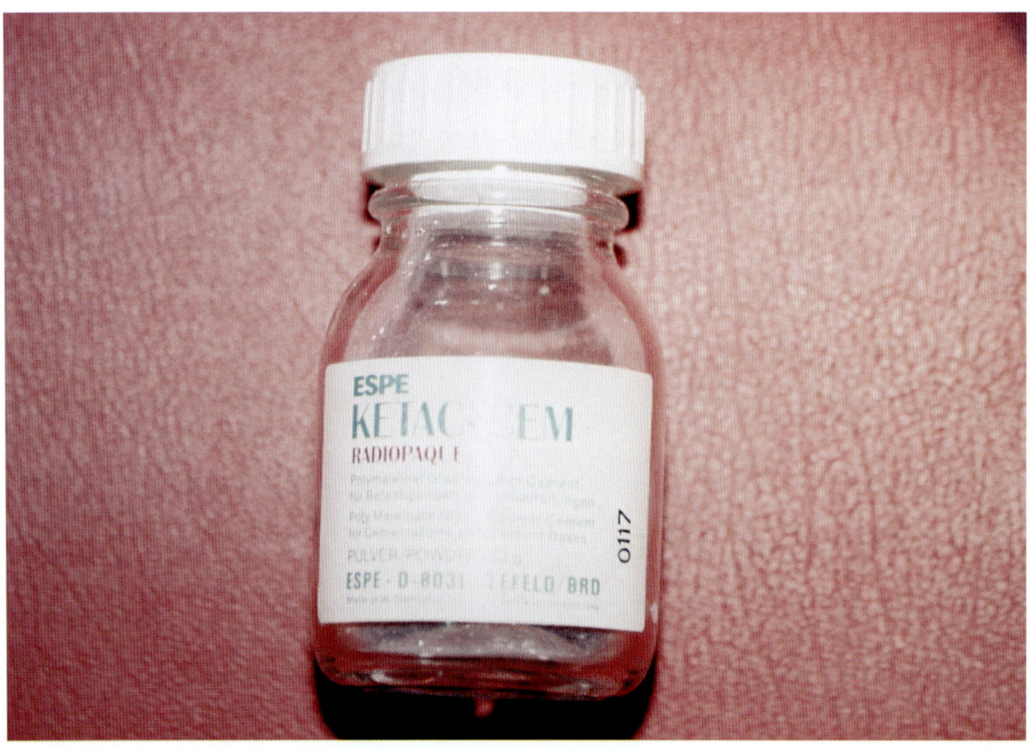

Fig 6–5. Glass ionomer cement.

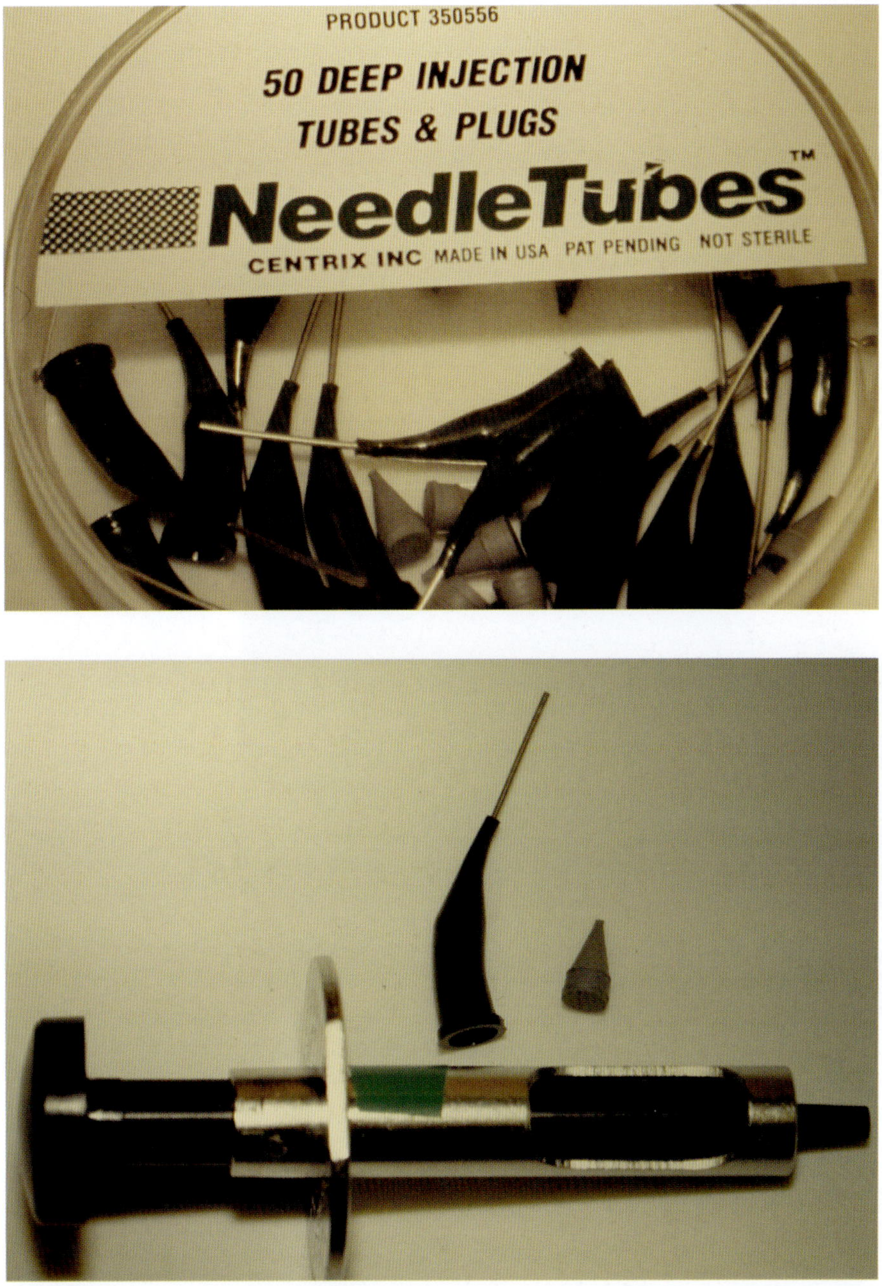

Fig 6–6A, B. Instrumentation utilized in performing a primary root canal.

alignment with the other teeth until a small bend is made in the supporting orthodontic wire.

Once the bands or crowns are fitted to the teeth, an impression of the dental arch is taken in alginate, and the model is poured including the bands or crowns. A 0.036-inch diameter stainless steel orthodontic wire is soldered as a backing for supporting the pontic teeth. Individual 0.016-supporting wires are soldered for support, and acrylic is used to attach the pediatric denture teeth to the appliance. A keyhole cut in the back of the denture tooth adds in its security. The color is generally one-half shade whiter than the adjacent teeth. Acrylic teeth discolor slightly and will match 6 months later. If an exact color match is chosen, the tooth will appear dirty in 6 months. It is not neces-

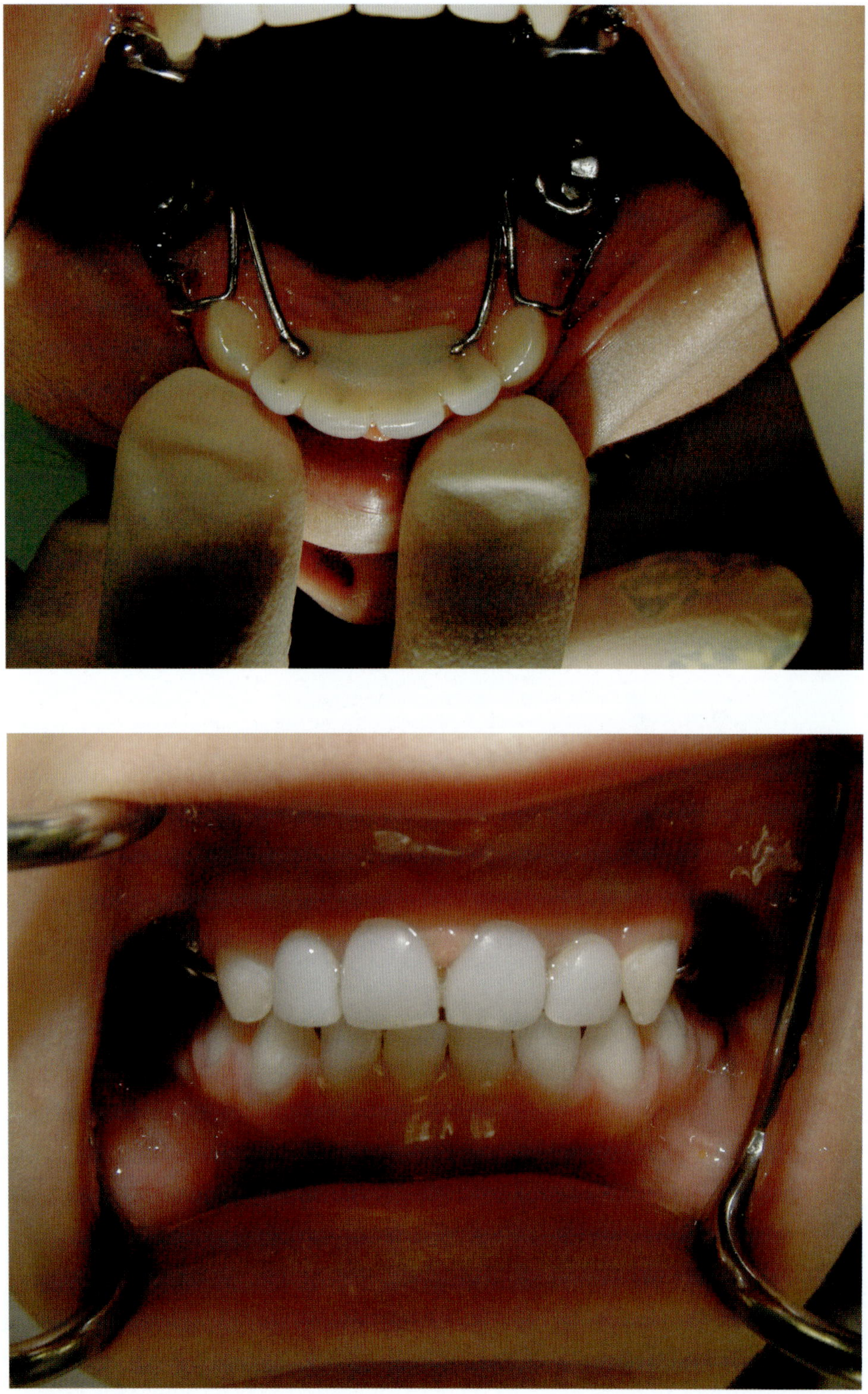

Fig 6–7A, B. Pediatric partial denture (Pedo-partial).

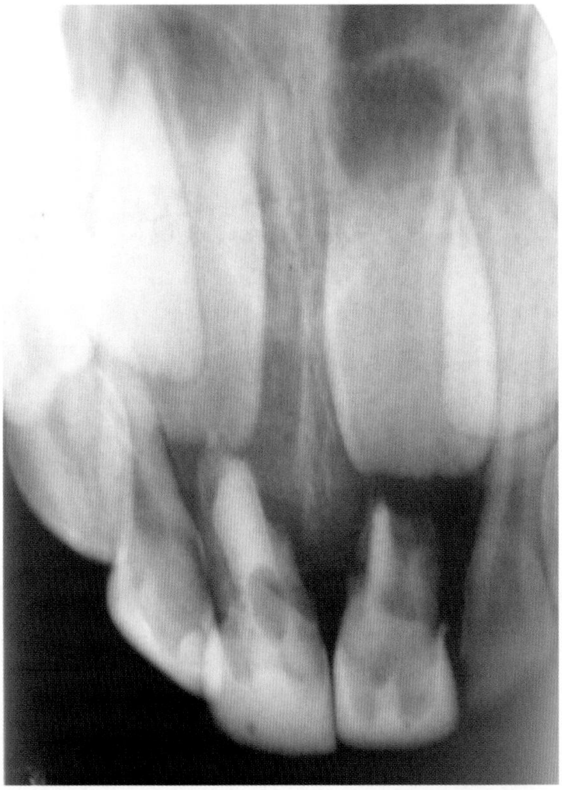

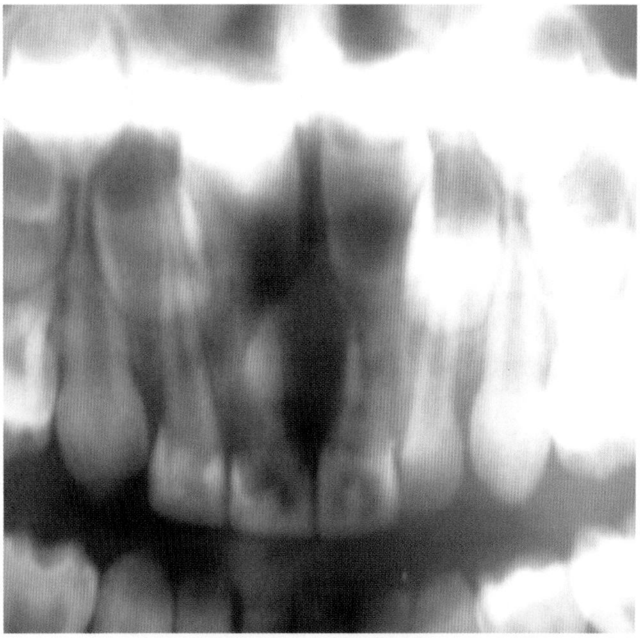

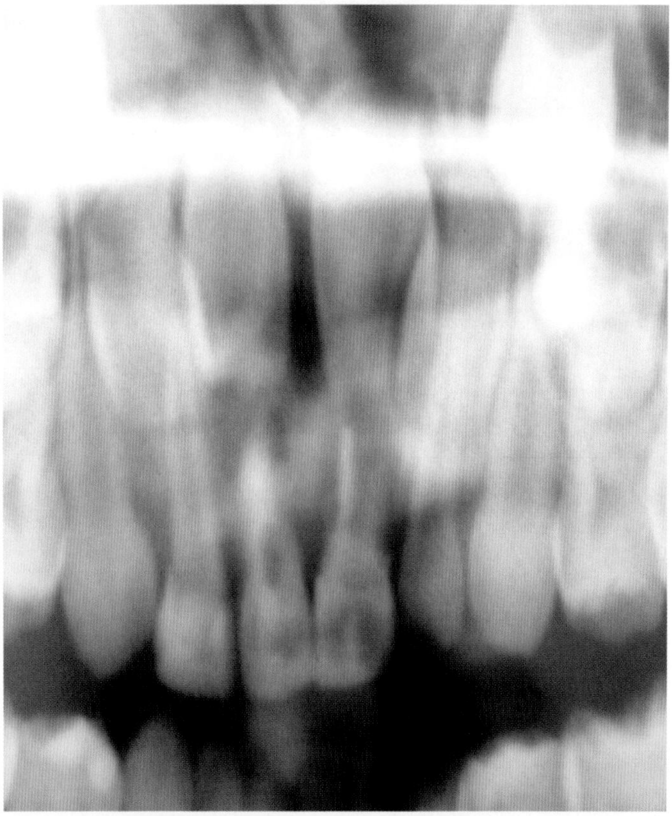

Fig 6–8A, B, C. Photos taken post-treated trauma.

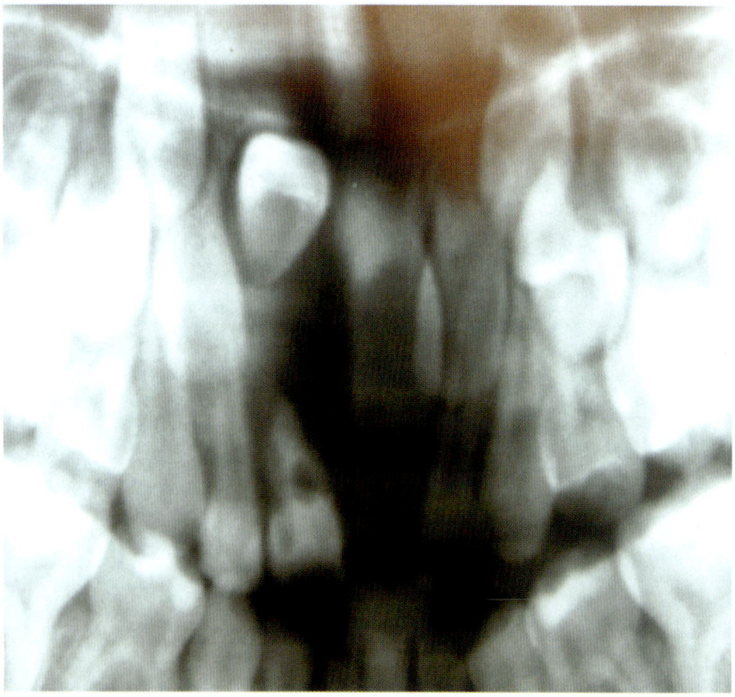

Fig 6–9. Right central incisor is displaced by traumatic bone cyst.

sary to add pink acrylic for the gum tissue. The esthetics will be much better if a tooth of the proper crown length of a 4-year-old child is used. Multiple teeth, including cuspid teeth, can be incorporated this way. If crowns are used, the 0.036-wire is cut with a high-speed bur at the mesial-lingual junction of the crown, and the crown can exfoliate with the eruption of the permanent bicuspid tooth.

These prosthetic replacements restore the function of the missing teeth. They also restore the proper morphology of the dental arch for proper speech development, and restore the morphology for proper swallowing pattern. In addition, these replacements maintain the space available for the eruption of the permanent teeth, and maintain the esthetics that were present prior to the injury.

FOLLOW-UP CARE FOR TRAUMA TO THE PRIMARY TEETH

There is a tendency to forget that a traumatic event has been sustained once the area has successfully healed and the child is a year older. Unfortunately, internal and external resorption is visible only with the proper radiograph. The area should be radiographed on an annual basis. The primary concern is the development of the permanent incisor tooth. Often, the eruption of the permanent incisor can be altered when the erupting tooth encounters denser alveolar bone, compacted or sclerosed by the traumatic incident years prior to the date of eruption. Chronic infection or irritation can cause enamel hypoplasia (bright white spot) on the permanent incisor, or alter the shape of the developing tooth. In a worst case scenario, a traumatic bone cyst can form apically to the primary teeth, and displace the permanent tooth bud under the patient's nose. It can also invert the crown so that the incisal edge points superiorly. These malposed incisor teeth do not require extraction; however, the orthodontic repositioning requires multiple surgical repositionings during the course of treatment. For some unexplained reason, the root on these teeth did not grow until the tooth was rotated orthodontically and well on its way into position in the three cases this author has treated.

TRAUMA TO THE PERMANENT DENTITION: AGES 6 TO 18 YEARS

There are significant differences in the approach to trauma for the permanent dentition. These differences are par-

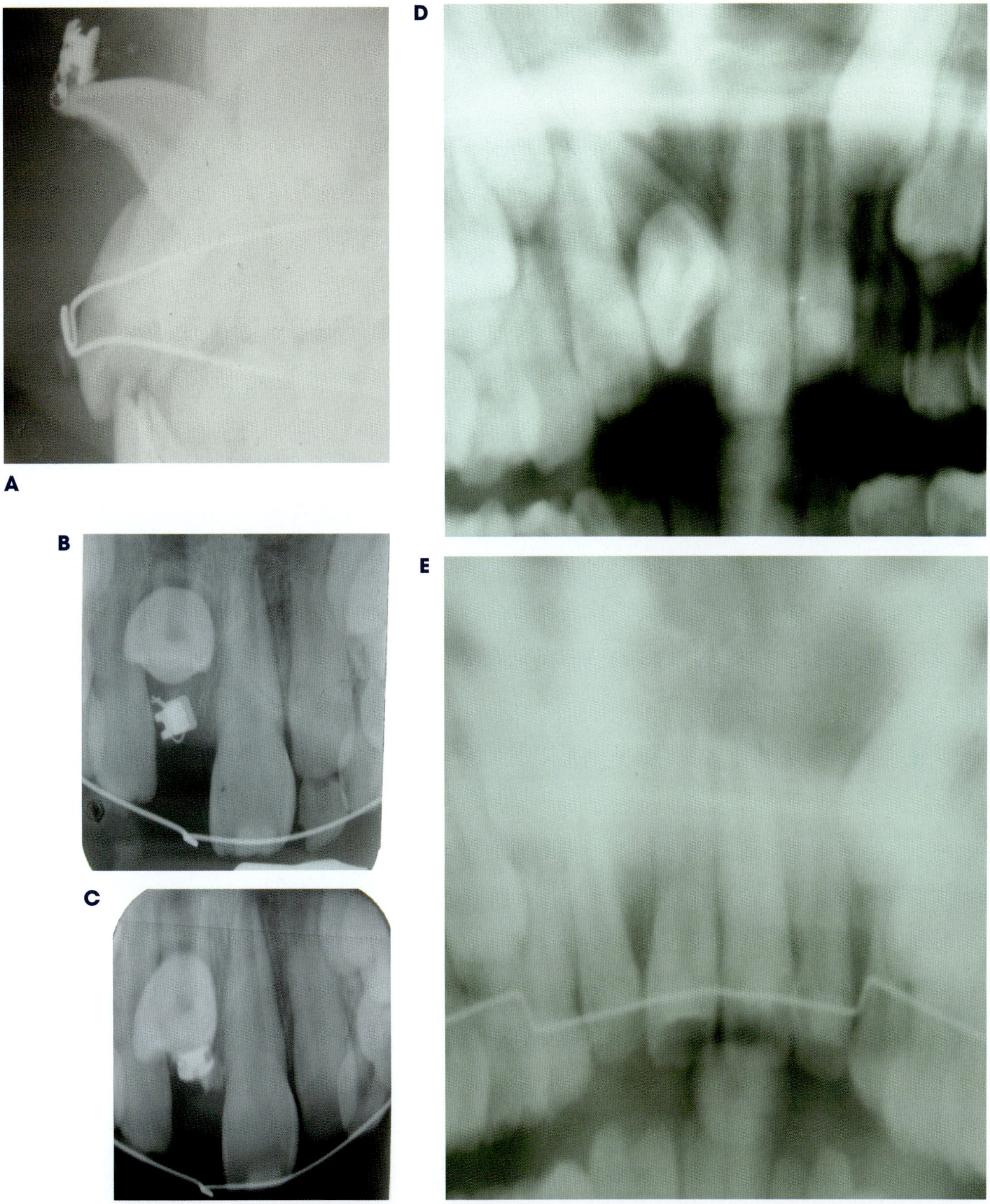

Fig 6–10A, B, C, D, E. Orthodontic realignment (A–D) post-trauma (Fig 6–8 and 6–9) with excellent results (E).

ticularly important when it comes to the stabilization of subluxated teeth, avulsed teeth, and fractured teeth when pulpal involvement occurs in immaturely developed teeth.

BLEEDING AROUND THE GUM TISSUE

Bleeding around the gum tissue is indicative of damage to the periodontal ligament, or the surrounding mucosal structures. Radiographs should be taken within 24 hours to check for root fracture, alveolar fracture, or mandibular fractures if no apparent displacement is initially noted. Proper antibiotic coverage should begin to prevent infection traveling down the periodontal ligament into the pulp tissue.

FRACTURED PERMANENT TOOTH

Most dentists are well versed and well equipped to restore fractured permanent teeth. First, the extent of the fracture is established. If bleeding comes from the center of the tooth, a direct pulp exposure has ensued. Calcium hydroxide is generally used to help build a dentin bridge in the healing process, followed by a copal varnish or glass ionomer cement for stability of this "Band-Aid." The tooth can later be repaired with composite restorative material. Rebonding the fractured part of the tooth may be satisfactory for a short-term repair, but they rarely last more than a few years before the bond fails and a restoration is required.

Fractures that occur horizontally below the crest of the alveolar bone have been known to heal with a "callous" formation around the injury. Stabilization of these teeth may be necessary. Vertical fractures that are below the crestal bone may later require orthodontic extrusion to allow proper restoration.[6]

When a permanent tooth erupts into the mouth, its root structure is not completely formed. It often takes 2 additional years for the root apex to close. Technically, it is difficult to endodontically treat the immature tooth because there is no stop for the filling material, and it may simply extrude out the apex of the tooth. Therefore, on these teeth it may be necessary to pack calcium hydroxide to build a calcium bridge so a stop can be fabricated. These teeth may require multiple packing attempts. The root does not continue to grow, and the treated tooth may have a shorter root than its contralateral counterpart.[7,8]

SUBLUXATED TOOTH

Teeth that are displaced from their original position require immediate repositioning if more than a few millimeters of displacement has occurred. Teeth that are invulsed but have remained stable, may be observed for their movement back to the original position. If they are not visible clinically, they may require surgical exposure, an orthodontic attachment placed on the crown of the tooth, and the tooth erupted orthodontically. One should not be tempted to reposition these with a forceps. If the crown has been knocked lingually, and the posterior teeth do not occlude due to the position of the incisor tooth, repositioning requires an extractionlike motion, followed by proper angulation, and repositioning to the original position. Stabilization of these teeth is required, and is discussed in the next section.

AVULSED TOOTH

When a permanent tooth is knocked out of the mouth, time is of the essence for reimplantation to occur. The tooth must be kept moist. The glycoprotein of milk is best, but if it is not readily available, a damp towel will serve well. The tooth should not be cleaned by untrained individuals, for the periodontal ligaments may be scrubbed off. Reimplantation within an hour of the injury has a 90%+ success rate. Delay of 3 hours decreases the odds down to 65% success. Soaking the tooth in Hanks solution (Fig 6–11), or the storage medium for organ transplantation will rehydrate the ligaments and greatly improve the success rate.

Very few of these injuries occur during office hours. Most require treatment in a hospital emergency room setting where suction and lighting is not optimal for placing orthodontic brackets for stabilization. Once the area has been anesthetized with a local anesthetic, a temporary splint can be easily fabricated in 15 minutes in the presence of blood and saliva that is commonly found in lacerated oral structures. First, a section of Eric arch bar material (Fig 6–12) is bent to match the curvature of the dentition. Its length extends at least three teeth on both sides of the avulsed teeth. Then a large amount of glass ionomer cement is mixed and placed on the smooth side of the arch bar. The teeth are then replaced and the arch bar laid on the teeth. The teeth are held with the fingers and thumbs until the cement sets (3–5 minutes). This

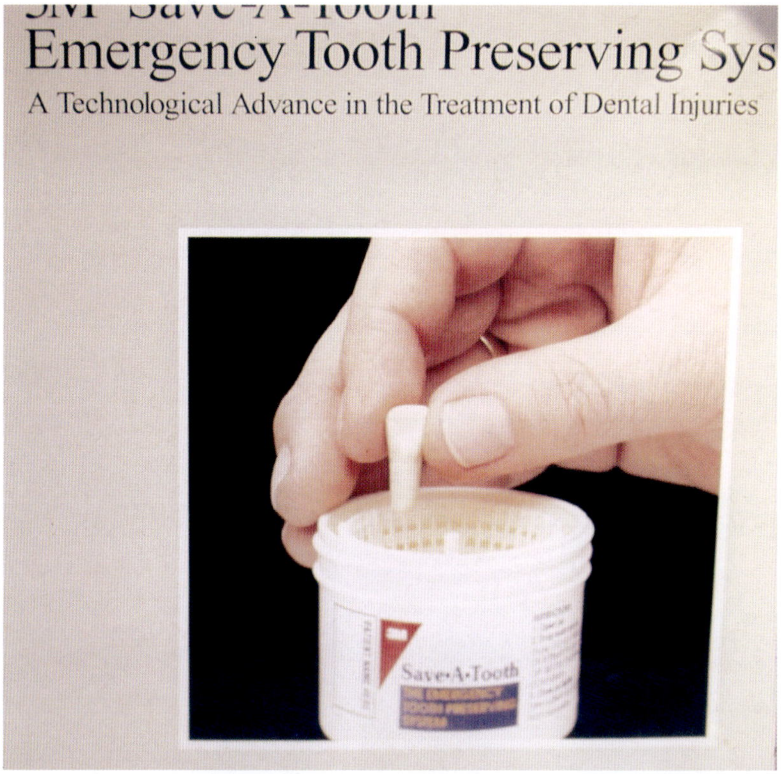

Fig 6–11. Hanks solution for rehydrating permanent incisors for reimplantation.

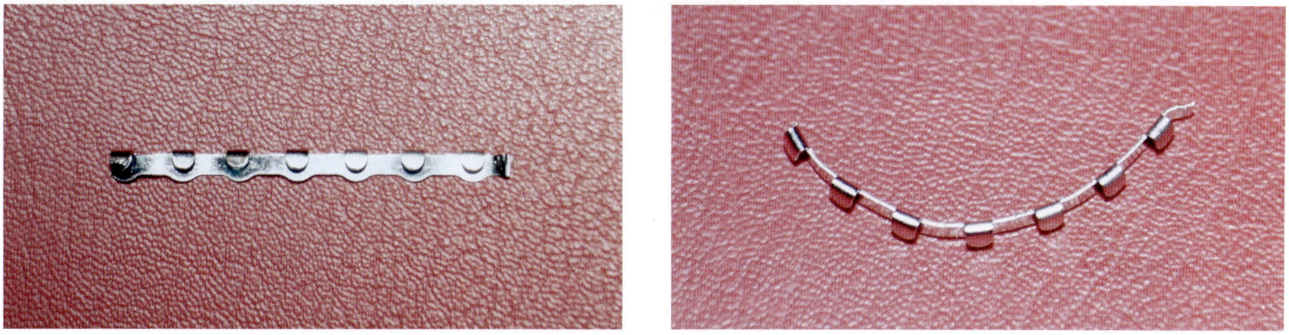

A **B**

Fig 6–12A, B. Eric arch bars.

gives a weak stabilization. Glass ionomer cements give off acid as they set and slightly etch the teeth. A dry field is not necessary. Then another large amount of cement is mixed and applied to the teeth and arch bar so a broad surface area is included. The loops on the arch bar hold the cement in place, and once the cement is dry (Fig 6–13), the patient is given antibiotics and analgesics and dismissed. Two days later, when the swelling has reduced and the patient is rested, the patient can be seen in the office, sedated with versed, the area anesthetized with a local anesthetic, and the arch bar and cement removed (Figure 6–14) with a high-speed rotary instrument. Orthodontic brackets are applied to the teeth and a light round wire is used to stabilize the teeth (Fig 6–15). Endodontic treatment is started at this visit, where the memory of the patient will be foggy at best. Most metropolitan hospitals have pediatric dentists and oral surgeons on staff who can be called to initiate and direct the proper treatment.

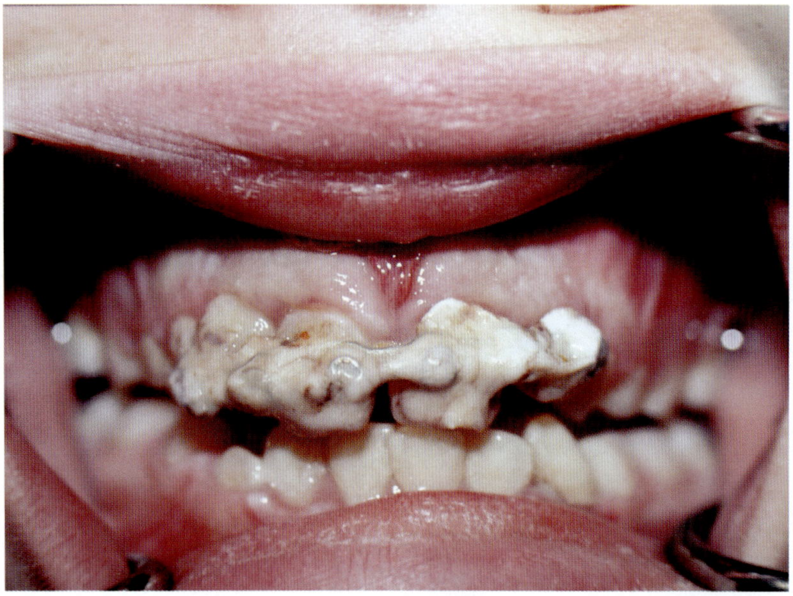

A

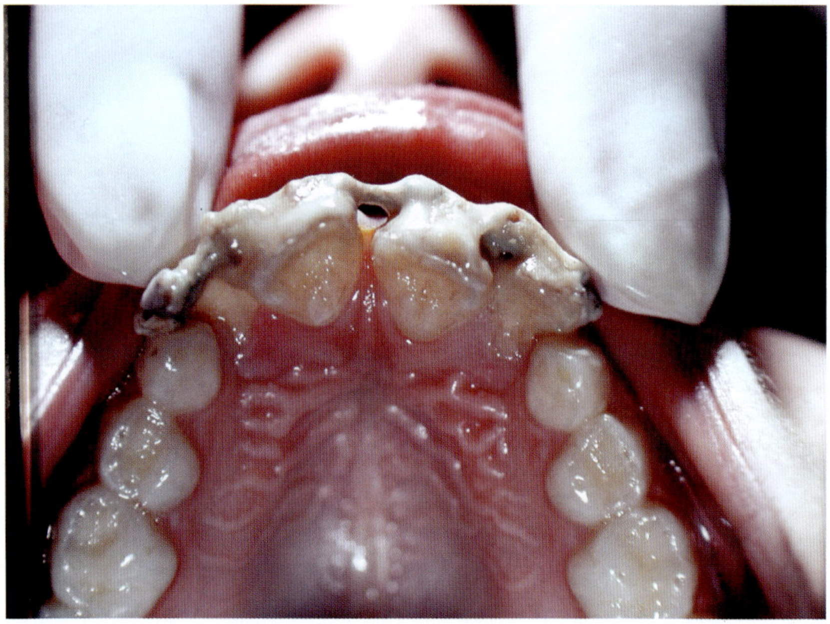

B

Fig 6–13A, B. Photos immediately poststabilization.

FOLLOW-UP TREATMENT

The two most frequent sequelae of failed treatment are pulpal necrosis with internal or external resorption, and ankylosis of the tooth to the bone. Endodontists are the dental specialists best equipped to retreat a failed traumatic injury to the tooth. Unfortunately, there are no good answers for an ankylosed tooth. Ankylosis takes the clinical appearance of the tooth submerging below the level of the adjacent teeth. Actually, these teeth do not submerge, but they are fused to the alveolar bone, and as the bone grows, the tooth remains in its original position. As the bone grows downward and forward, the tooth appears to sink into the gum tissue. Surgical repositioning of the tooth in a growing child has a high incidence of reankylosing. These teeth do not move orthodontically.

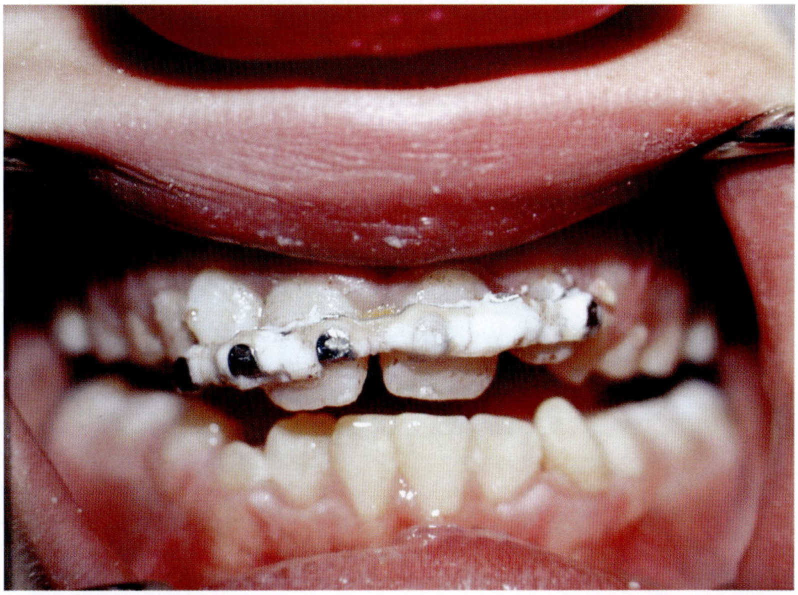

Fig 6–14. Photo demonstrating removal of cement.

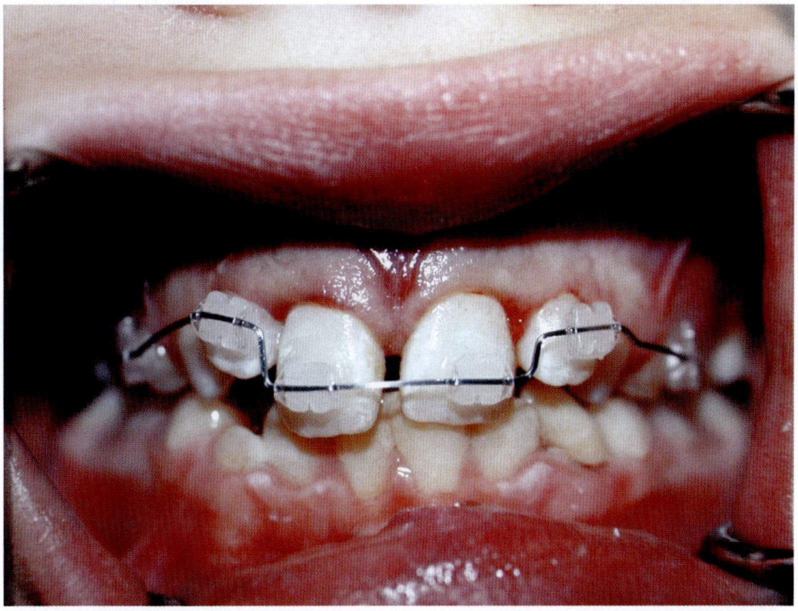

Fig 6–15. Orthodontic bracelets placed in the office setting.

Ankylosis interferes with the developing alveolar bone, so over-retention of these teeth may leave a defect that may not adequately support a dental implant. All the dental disciplines that will be treating the patient should be consulted when deciding the best course of treatment. Maxillary sutures can also ankylose, leaving a situation where one side of the maxillae grows downward faster than the other, leaving one central incisor tooth longer and a posterior unilateral open bite. A surgical down-fracture may be necessary once the patient stops growing. Temporary replacement for a missing permanent tooth can include an orthodontic retainer with a pontic, a bleaching tray with a pontic, a ribbond, or Maryland bridge attached to the lingual of the adjacent teeth. Dental implants along with prosthetic replacements are the best long-term replacements. Even the best of crowns only last 20 to 25 years and will require replacement. This should be taken into account when medical accident insurance claims or liability tort are calculated.

PREVENTION

As the old saying goes, an ounce of prevention is worth a pound of cure. Mouth guards and helmets should be worn when potentially dangerous activities are played. Class II malocclusions that are maxillary protrusive in nature should receive interceptive orthodontic therapy at age 8 to retract the front teeth out of the "fracture zone." Multiple children on a single trampoline are dangerous—an accident waiting to happen. Rollerblades and skateboards should be limited to areas designated for those sports. Bicycles require maintenance that includes making sure handles and seats remain secure, and the tires are properly inflated.

REFERENCES

1. Andreasen JO. *Traumatic Injuries of the Teeth.* 2nd ed. Copenhagen: Munksgaard:1981.
2. Cassamassimo Paul S. In critical condition: management of dental trauma. *J Ped Dent.* 1995;17(5):330–331.
3. Kenny DJ. Recent developments in dental traumatology. *J Ped Dent.* 2001;23(6):464–468.
4. Lombadi S, Sheller B, Willeams B. Diagnosis and treatment of dental trauma in a children's hospital. *J Ped Dent.* 1998;20(2):112–120.
5. Merkle A. Complete intrusion of a maxillary right primary central incisor. *J Ped Dent.* 2000;22(2):151–152.
6. Sweet CA. A classification and treatment for traumatized anterior teeth. *J Dent Children.* 1955;22:144–149.
7. Down CH. The treatment of permanent incisor teeth for children following traumatic injury. *Aust Dent J.* 1957;2:9–24.
8. Hargreaves, JA. Emergency treatment for injuries to anterior teeth. *Int Dent J.* 1974;24:18–29.

7

Frontal Sinus Fractures and Neurosurgical Issues in Pediatric Trauma

Carrie R. Muh
David M. Wrubel

INTRODUCTION

Children suffer approximately 5% of maxillofacial trauma.[1] Two to twelve percent of craniofacial traumas involve frontal sinus fractures.[2-4] When evaluated and managed properly, pediatric patients with frontal sinus fractures generally have a good outcome. However, serious complications can arise and these patients do require both acute evaluation and long-term follow-up. Although there are no strict guidelines for operative management, there have been several studies that can be used to guide treatment decisions.

ANATOMY

Although development of the frontal sinus ostium begins during the third or fourth month of gestation, the sinus itself is not present at birth. In utero, a furrow forms between the first and second ethmoturbinals, which will eventually form the frontal recess.[5,6] Primary pneumatization of the frontal sinus occurs in utero; however, the sinus remains without significant further development until a child is approximately 2 years old at which time secondary pneumatization occurs.[5] Anterior ethmoid infundibular air cells invade the frontal bone through the frontal recess or superior meatus and this pneumatization extends vertically upward over the next decade or more.[6]

By 3 years of age, the pneumatized area extends to just above the nasion. By approximately 6 years of age, the pneumatized sinus reaches the frontal bone and becomes radiographically visible.[1,7] The sinus does not extend above the roof of the orbits until roughly 8 years of age, and it continues to expand in size until late adolescence at 12 to 15 years of age. It is the last of the sinuses to form and is quite variable from one person to another. The frontal sinuses are often asymmetric, and a hypoplastic sinus can be found in up to 20% of patients.[3,5,8] In 4% of the population, at least one sinus is entirely unformed.[5,6] Because of this late development, fractures through the sinus are not seen in small children. The fully formed adult sinus is a rather small pyramidal shape, with a volume of approximately 5 to 7 mL and average dimensions of 2.4 cm high, 2.9 cm wide, and 2.0 cm deep.[5]

The anterior wall of the sinus contains cancellous as well as cortical bone and is significantly thicker and tougher than the posterior wall. The posterior table is generally tightly adherent to the dura. The horizontal portion of the frontal bone that forms the roof of the orbit is the thinnest wall of the sinus.[5] A more pneumatized sinus will consist of thinner bone and will therefore have an increased risk of injury with trauma.

In the posteromedial aspect of the sinus floor is the nasofrontal duct, the drainage foramen for the frontal sinus.[6] A true duct is present in only 15% of sinuses, whereas up to 85% lack a true duct and the sinuses drain through air cells into the middle meatus.[5] When present, the duct has a variable route and can run caudally for a few millimeters or up to 2 cm.

The arterial supply to the frontal sinus is provided by the anterior ethmoidal branch of the internal carotid artery and often the supraorbital branch of the ophthalmic artery. A branch off the supraorbital artery supplies the diploe of the frontal bone and may continue to the mucoperiosteum of the sinus. Venous drainage occurs through multiple small diploic veins of Breschet which travel through small mucosa-lined foramina in the cortical bone. These small veins drain to the dural venous sinuses as well as the frontal diploic vein, which then joins the supraorbital vein to form the superior ophthalmic vein and empties into the cavernous sinus.[5] The ophthalmic veins do not contain valves and may permit infection to spread from a frontal sinus fracture to the cavernous sinus. Infection may also travel via the veins of Breschet to the dural sinuses.

The mucosal lining of the frontal sinus consists of pseudostratified ciliated columnar epithelium and is contiguous with the mucosa of the nasofrontal ducts and ethmoid air cells as well as the foramina of Breschet.

Parasympathetic innervation to the mucosal glands comes from the lateral superior posterior nasal nerves via the pterygopalatine ganglion after originating in the superior salivatory nucleus. The pterygopalatine ganglion also provides sympathetic fibers to the mucosa. Sensation to the mucosa comes from the anterior ethmoidal branch of the nasociliary nerve as well as supraorbital and supratrochlear branches of the frontal nerve. Frontal sinusitis may therefore cause pain at the forehead and the anterior fossa dura.

PRESENTATION

Frontal sinus fractures represent 2 to 12% of facial trauma.[2-4] The most common causes of frontal sinus fractures in children are motor vehicle accidents and all-terrain vehicle accidents. The anterior table can withstand a force of 800 to 2200 pounds before it will fracture.[1,6] This is significantly higher than that which other facial bones can tolerate and therefore it is common for a patient to have additional injuries. Up to 95% of patients with frontal sinus fractures present with multiple facial or skull fractures,[8,7] and 35 to 64% of pediatric patients have an associated intracranial injury.[1,7,9] Younger patients have an increased risk of associated intracranial injury than do adults.[10] This may be due to the lower rate of pneumatization in a child's skull causing a larger transfer of forces to the skull base and intracranial vault, or to the higher craniofacial ratio in a young child, which decreases with age.[1]

Frontal sinus fractures should be considered whenever a laceration, abrasion, or ecchymosis is seen at the inferior forehead, supraorbital ridge, or glabella. This is the most common clinical finding.[11] Patients may also present with cerebrospinal fluid (CSF) rhinorrhea, forehead anesthesia, anosmia, or visual changes. Due to the nature of the injury, patients may present comatose or with orthopedic, abdominal, or thoracic injuries as well.

WORKUP

A full physical exam is necessary to assess for other injuries. Ophthalmologic evaluation may be needed to assess vision and extraocular movements in the setting of an orbital fracture.

Roentgenograms (x-rays) have traditionally been used to diagnose frontal sinus fractures. The sensitivity is not very high for smaller or nondisplaced fractures, however, and x-rays often do not provide significant information on damage to the midface or the posterior table. Now that computed tomography (CT) scans are easily accessible at most trauma centers, this is the recommended radiologic imaging. The sensitivity is considerably higher than with x-rays and CT permits concomitant evaluation of the intracranial structures as well as the midface. The nasofrontal duct cannot be clearly visualized on most CT scans; however, injury to the duct is suggested when there is injury to the base of the sinus or the ethmoids.[11] Whereas axial views will give a good assessment of the anterior and posterior walls, coronal reconstructions should also be obtained to provide additional information about the condition of the sinus roof and floor, the nasofrontal ducts, and injury to the orbit and other facial bones.[1,12]

HISTORY

Many different operations on the frontal sinus have been described over the past two centuries. Runge performed obliteration of the frontal sinus as early as 1750.[13,14] In 1884, Ogston described trephination of the anterior wall with preservation of nasal drainage, and Schonborn developed an osteoplastic flap for access to the frontal sinus in 1894.[14,15] The first ablative procedure for a frontal sinus fracture was described by Reidel in 1898 when he removed the anterior table and sinus floor allowing the skin to lie over the posterior table.[15,16] In 1904, Killian attempted to improve the cosmetic result of this procedure by leaving a rim of supraorbital bone intact.[14] Lynch described the frontoethmoidectomy in 1921 when he removed the sinus floor and ethmoids, but left the anterior table intact and inserted a drain from the sinus to the nose.[15,17] The next advancements were made in 1951 and 1955 when Bergara improved the osteoplastic flap procedure by removing the anterior table but leaving it hinged to a piece of pericranium to provide an improved cosmetic result.[16,17] In 1958, Goodale and Montgomery advanced the osteoplastic flap procedure further by removing all the sinus mucosa then packing it off with fat.[14] This was a definite improvement; however, failure to remove all the mucosa led to mucocele or mucopyocele. Donald and Bernstein took the surgical treatment of frontal sinus fractures a step further with cranialization of the sinus in 1978.[17] The entire posterior table was removed, the sinus mucosa was stripped, the nasofrontal ducts were plugged with fat, and the brain was allowed to expand into the sinus cavity. This procedure is still in use for patients with displaced posterior wall fractures.

Multiple operative options exist today, ranging from minimally invasive to full cranialization. The major factor in deciding which procedure to pursue is the type of fracture present.

CLASSIFICATION

Although numerous classification schemes have been presented, most authors classify fractures simply by location and severity. Three structures must be considered: the anterior table, posterior table, and nasofrontal duct.[9,11,18] Fractures may affect the anterior table, the posterior table, or both. They may be simple (Fig 7–1) or comminuted (Figs 7–2 and 7–3), displaced or nondisplaced, open or

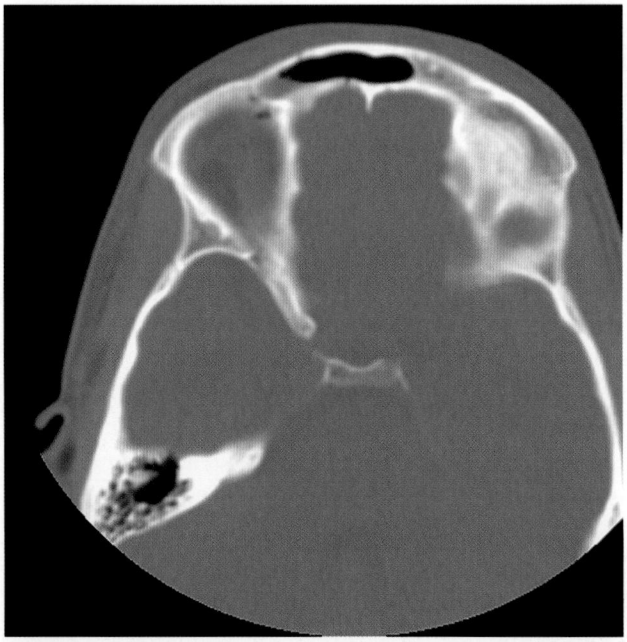

Fig 7–1. Simple, nondisplaced fracture involving the anterior and posterior table of the frontal sinus.

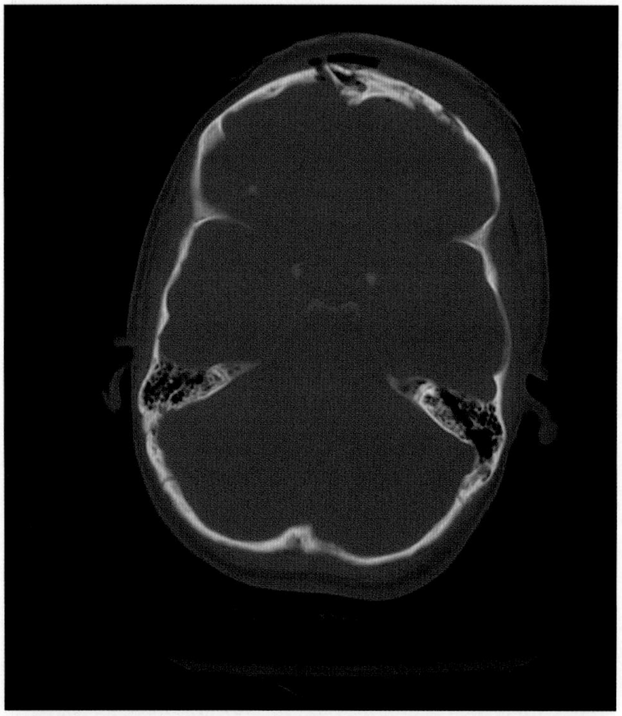

Fig 7–2. Comminuted fracture involving the frontal sinus.

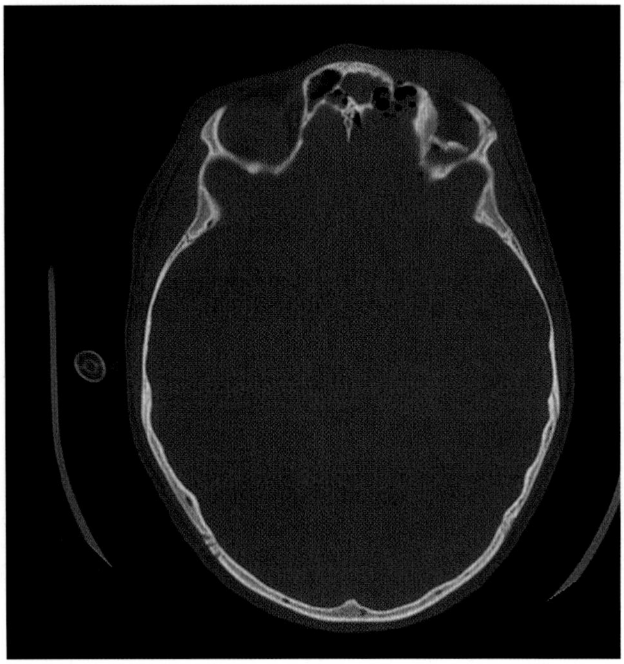

Fig 7–3. Fracture involving the frontal sinus and left orbit.

closed. They may involve obvious CSF leak, an open laceration, or an open cerebral injury.

Isolated posterior table fractures are quite rare, whereas isolated anterior table fractures are the most common form of frontal sinus fracture, comprising up to 72% of frontal sinus fractures.[2] Anterior wall fractures can lead to blockage of the duct as well as cosmetic deformities. Posterior wall fractures may result in direct cerebral injury, dural laceration and CSF leak, mucocele formation, or infection including abscess or meningitis.

MANAGEMENT

Management decisions should be based on the type of fracture present. Closed, nondisplaced isolated anterior wall fractures should be managed with conservative monitoring and cosmetic evaluation once edema resolves. If fluid is seen within the sinus and does not clear on delayed repeat imaging, then the patient should be evaluated for possible nasofrontal ostia occlusion or CSF leak.[19] Open fractures require exploration of the laceration for debris as well as closure of the laceration. Anterior wall fractures that are displaced further than the width of the cortical plate will generally require fixation to restore facial aesthetics, and severely comminuted anterior wall fractures may require exenteration of the sinus. The nasofrontal duct should also be evaluated intraoperatively to assess for occlusion. If there is a large forehead laceration, this can be used to provide surgical access; however, more often, a bicoronal incision is utilized.

The treatment of closed, nondisplaced posterior wall fractures remains more controversial.[19,20] These should be evaluated for CSF leak or pneumocephalus but can often be treated conservatively with observation. Some authors recommend operative repair of any CSF leak, whereas others support a more conservative approach allowing the leak to resolve spontaneously. This has been based on the realization that there may be an increased number of complications relating from surgery than would have occurred by observing the fracture.[20] Displaced posterior wall fractures generally require operative exploration of the dura and nasofrontal duct as well as possible cranialization of the sinus with removal of entire mucosal lining and closure of anterior wall.

The treatment options available to surgically manage frontal sinus fractures have been expanding. Previously, craniotomy was the dominant treatment method. This usually necessitates a bicoronal incision. A bifrontal craniotomy is then performed. The posterior wall of the sinus is removed, commonly with bone rongeurs. The dura is inspected for any lacerations, which are primarily repaired. The mucosa is stripped from the sinus and the nasofrontal duct is occluded by packing, either with previously harvested bone fragments or another occlusive material. The sinus can be packed with any number of materials including Gelfoam, fat, muscle, or one of the newer hydroxyapatite cements. A pericranial flap is commonly used to create another layer of isolation between the cranial contents and the nasal passages. After the pericranial graft has been suspended, the anterior wall is reconstructed and the frontal bone is reattached using a plating system. The incision is then closed in layers.

Recently, some authors have advocated a less invasive endoscopic approach,[21] which can be accomplished with two small incisions behind the hairline. This technique can be used either to repair the fracture in the acute stage or to provide cosmesis with a depressed fracture in a delayed fashion.

COMPLICATIONS AND OTHER NEUROSURGICAL CONCERNS

Many complications are associated with frontal sinus fractures ranging from life threatening to very minor. The most worrisome complication is CSF leak, generally presenting as rhinorrhea. Up to 36% of patients with frontal sinus fractures will develop a CSF leak.[1,9] CSF rhinorrhea can occur immediately after the injury or in a delayed fashion. CSF rhinorrhea necessitates surgical intervention to decrease the likelihood of developing meningitis. Exploration and repair of the dura are usually indicated to stop the CSF rhinorrhea; however, many clinicians will attempt lumbar drainage prior to surgery to allow the leak to heal. This does entail the separate risk of pneumocephalus in the presence of a large defect. Also, there is an increased amount of time during which meningitis may develop.

In any patient with CSF rhinorrhea due to a frontal sinus fracture, meningitis is an overriding concern. This provides an impetus to intervene quickly. Prior to intervention, the use of prophylactic antibiotics has been a matter of significant controversy. There have been no single studies that have definitively decided the matter.[22] Treatment with prophylactic antibiotics generally varies greatly between practitioners; however, meta-analysis of the literature does seem to support a role for prophylactic antibiotics in the presence of CSF rhinorrhea after a traumatic event.[22,23] Development of meningitis does necessitate a significant period of treatment. Patients with frontal sinus fractures are at risk for other infectious complications requiring treatment as well, including abscess formation, frontal sinusitis, and osteomyelitis.[17,20]

Delayed complications can arise after a frontal sinus injury. Poor cosmesis at the fracture site is the least serious medically, but can be a source of significant concern on the part of the patient. A potentially more serious, delayed complication is mucocele formation. This can result in significant mass effect on the frontal lobes and increase the risk of delayed meningitis. Mucoceles can form from blockage of the nasofrontal duct or from residual sinus mucosa after a cranialization procedure. Mucocele formation requires operative intervention for resection and repair.

In addition to the sequela of the frontal sinus fracture itself, other injuries can be associated with pediatric craniofacial trauma. Up to 10% of patients with frontal sinus fractures have associated epidural hematomas[9,24] or subdural hematomas,[1] and 25 to 55% have associated intraparenchymal hemorrhages or contusions.[1,24] Between 2.5 and 13% of patients with frontal sinus fractures present with open cerebral wounds.[9,24]

The majority of patients with frontal fractures suffer other facial or skull fractures as well, including orbital, nasal, and temporal fractures. These have their own related complications including diplopia, anosmia, CSF otorrhea, hearing loss, and facial nerve palsies.[4,25]

"Growing skull fractures" or leptomeningeal cysts are rare entities that form in less than 1% of childhood skull fractures.[26,27] More than 90% occur in children under the age of 3 years, with half occurring in children under the age of 1 year.[26,28] The majority of these fractures are located at the site of linear fractures in the frontal or parietal region. Although the pathogenesis is not fully understood, they are thought to be due to a tear in the dura of a growing brain. The pulsatile force of the rapidly growing brain causes an erosion of the bone edges and diastasis of the fracture line whereas underlying parenchymal or dural injury leads to arachnoid adhesions.[27,28] Together, these lead to a palpable skull defect with a local cyst that generally presents weeks to months after the traumatic event and requires surgical repair.

CONCLUSION

Frontal sinus fractures, although not the most common skull fracture in children, do occur with some regularity. Management of these fractures, although still under some debate, does require a combined specialty approach. Recent advances in endoscopic procedures and nonoperative management of more types of fractures can result in better outcomes and lower cost associated with this type of injury.

REFERENCES

1. Whatley WS, Allison DW, Chandra RK, et al. Frontal sinus fractures in children. *Laryngoscope.* 2005;115:1741–1745.
2. El Khatib K, Danino A, Malka G. The frontal sinus: a culprit or a victim? A review of 40 cases. *J Craniomaxillofac Surg.* 2004;32:314–317.
3. Gonty AA, Marciani RD, Adornato DC. Management of frontal sinus fractures. *J Oral Maxillofac Surg.* 1999; 57:372–379; discussion 380–381.

4. Sailer HF, Grätz KW, Kalavrezos ND. Frontal sinus fractures: principles of treatment and long-term results after sinus obliteration with the use of lyophilized cartilage. *J Craniomaxillofac Surg.* 1998;26(4):235–242.
5. McLaughlin RB Jr, Rehl RM, Lanza DC. Clinically relevant frontal sinus anatomy and physiology. *Otolaryngol Clin North Am.* 2001; 34:1–22.
6. Manolidis S. Management of frontal sinus trauma. *Sem Plast Surg.* 2002; 16(3):261–271.
7. Wright DL, Hoffman HT, Hoyt DB. Frontal sinus fractures in the pediatric population. *Laryngoscope.* 1992; 102(11):1215–1219.
8. Ginsburg CM. Frontal sinus fractures. *Pediatr Rev.* 1997; 18(4):120–121.
9. Gerbino G, Roccia F, Benech A, Caldarelli C. Analysis of 158 frontal sinus fractures: current surgical management and complications. *J Craniomaxillofac Surg.* 2000; 28(3):133–139.
10. McGraw BL, Cole RR. Pediatric maxillofacial trauma: age-related variations in injury. *Arch Otolaryngol Head Neck Surg.* 1990;116:41–45.
11. Harris L, Marano GD, McCorkle D. Nasofrontal duct: CT in frontal sinus trauma. *Radiology.* 1987;165(1):195–198.
12. Tanrikulu R, Erol B. Comparison of computed tomography with conventional radiography for midfacial fractures. *Dentomaxillofac Radiol.* 2001;30(3):141–146.
13. Meyer TK, Smith TL. Contemporary issues in frontal sinus surgery. *Curr Opin Otolaryngol Head Neck Surg.* 2002;10:8–13.
14. Lawson W, Reino AJ. Management of embossment following the frontal osteoplastic operation. *Laryngoscope.* 1996;106:1259–1265.
15. Seiden AM, Stankiewicz JA. Frontal sinus surgery: the state of the art. *Am J Otolaryngol.* 1998;19(3):183–193.
16. Manolidis S. Frontal sinus injuries: associated injuries and surgical management of 93 patients. *J Oral Maxillofac Surg.* 2004;62:882–891.
17. Bell RB, Dierks EJ, Brar P, Potter JK, Potter BE. A protocol for the management of frontal sinus fractures emphasizing sinus preservation. *J Oral Maxillofac Surg.* 2007;65(5):825–839.
18. Luce EA. Frontal sinus fractures: guidelines to management. *Plast Reconstr Surg.* 1987; 80(4):500–507.
19. Metzinger SE, Guerra AB, Garcia RE. Frontal sinus fractures: management guidelines. *Facial Plast Surg.* 2005; 21(3):199–206.
20. Gossman DG, Archer SM, Arosarena O. Management of frontal sinus fractures: a review of 96 cases. *Laryngoscope.* 2006;116(8):1357–1362.
21. Pham AM, Strong EB. Endoscopic management of facial fractures. *Curr Opin Otolaryngol Head Neck Surg.* 2006;14(4):234–241.
22. Brodie HA. Prophylactic antibiotics for posttraumatic cerebrospinal fluid fistulae: a meta-analysis. *Arch Otolaryngol Head Neck Surg.* 2006;123(7):749–752.
23. Friedman JA, Ebersold MJ, Quast LM. Persistent post-traumatic cerebrospinal fluid leakage. *Neurosurg Focus.* 2000;9(1):e1.
24. Strong EB, Pahlavan N, Saito D. Frontal sinus fractures: a 28-year retrospective review. *Otolaryngol Head Neck Surg.* 2006;135(5):774–779.
25. Lee D, Honrado C, Har-El G, Goldsmith A. Pediatric temporal bone fractures. *Laryngoscope.* 1998;108(6):816–821.
26. Suri A, Mahapatra AK. Growing fractures of the orbital roof. A report of two cases and a review. *Pediatr Neurosurg.* 2002;36(2):96–100.
27. Sugiultzoglu MK, Souweidane MM. Early management of craniocerebral injury with avoidance of post-traumatic leptomeningeal cyst formation. Report of two cases. *Pediatr Neurosurg.* 2001;35(6):329–333.
28. Ziyal IM, Aydin Y, Türkmen CS, et al. The natural history of late diagnosed or untreated growing skull fractures: report on two cases. *Acta Neurochir (Wien).* 1998; 140(7):651–654.

8

Injuries Related to Facial Growth and Fracture Patterns in Pediatric Trauma

Frederick Durden
Amanda Corey

It has been well documented that trauma is the most common cause of mortality and morbidity in childhood.[1] Each year 150,000 children are permanently disabled and 15,000 die as a result of trauma-related injuries.[2] In addition, trauma-related injuries are the leading cause of child hospitalizations.[3] Despite the high incidences of traumatic injury, facial bone fractures are uncommon in the pediatric group. This is due to developmental anatomy and the specific types of trauma. Because of the rare and diverse presentation of pediatric facial fractures, it is important to be vigilant in the recognition of these injuries and their potential complication so as to involve appropriate medical subspecialties early in the management process. This chapter aims to offer a foundation to understanding and treatment by discussing epidemiology, anatomic changes in relation to fracture pattern, and potential complications of pediatric facial fractures.

Facial growth is a complex process. The involvement of adjacent bone segments and soft tissue covering is needed to guide the facial structures into correct alignment.

Two of the more important dynamics to facial maturation are bony growth and sinus development. The cranium to facial ratio changes from 8:1 at birth to 2:1 during the second decade of life. The cranium reaches 80% of its final size by age 2. Because of this, the face is somewhat protected by the larger cranium at birth. This is highlighted by the higher incidence of cranium injuries in children particularly those less than 7 years of age as compared to the incidence of facial injuries.[4,5]

The contribution of the growth of the bony skeleton to facial development is a result of a process of absorption and deposition. This is under the guidance of soft tissue covering, which includes fascia, tendon, muscle, and skin. Growth results in bone movement by primary and secondary displacement. Primary displacement is a result of individual bone absorption and deposition. Secondary growth, however, is a product of the interrelation between different bony segments.[4] For example, the final position of the alveolar ridge is a result of both primary growth of the maxilla and secondarily to zygoma and orbital bone growth.

In addition to bony growth, sinus development also contributes to facial development and trauma patterns. At birth the sinuses are present as mucosal buds. Similar to facial growth, the sinuses develop by primary and secondary growth. Primary growth is the out-pouching of the mucosal buds. Secondary growth begins when pneumatization extends the early sinuses into the surrounding cartilaginous and bony structures. Maxillary sinus growth begins around the second fetal month. Secondary maxillary growth begins at the fifth month and continues to expand inferiorly and laterally until completion between the ages of 15 to18 years. It is important to remember that by the second year of life the maxillary sinus has extended to the infraorbital canal. This alters susceptibility to orbital fractures, which is discussed later. The frontal and ethmoid sinuses begin growth later during the fourth month of fetal development. The frontal sinuses are rarely radiographically visible until the seventh or eighth years of life. The sphenoid sinus differs from other sinuses, as its growth does not involve primary growth. Sphenoid growth begins with constriction of the sphenoethmoidal recess. This invagination is separated from the nasal cavity by mucosa, which later develops into cartilage. By the fifth year of life, the cartilage structure attaches to the sphenoid bone. Secondary sphenoid growth starts at age 7 and a radiographically visible sinus is present by age 10. As the sinuses enlarge, they offer some protection to the globe and intracranial structures. Also eruption of permanent teeth alters fracture patterns of the maxilla (Fig 8–1), as discussed later in this chapter.[6]

As previously stated, the development of the face is complex. It is obviously not possible to have prospective studies of facial growth changes and the effect this has on a traumatic injury profile. However, it is known that the changing ratio of cranium to face and the development of sinus all serve to place the facial skeleton in increasing risk of traumatic injury. The dependency of bony segments on one another for correct placement adds importance to recognition and management of pediatric facial trauma. It is important to recognize that incorrect repair or iatragenic disruption of growth plates can lead to increased morbidity of facial fractures.

PATTERNS OF FRACTURE

The etiology and strength of the traumatic event along with the anatomic features introduced above dictate the pattern of pediatric facial trauma. Mandibular fractures are the most common fracture in hospitalized children. The highest frequency corresponds to the condylar head. This is due to its thin neck and high vascularity. It is followed by the symphysis, angle, and body fractures, respectively.[7,8] Midface fractures in children increase as the sinuses evolve. Maxillary and nasal fractures are most common followed by zygoma fractures. It is thought that midface fractures in children are the result of higher impact forces. Despite this fact, Le Fort fractures are unusual particularly in children less than 2 years of age (Fig 8–2).[9,10] Orbital fractures are the result of direct force to the bony orbit and hydraulic effect of displaced orbital soft tissues. It has been shown that orbital floor fractures in children are more likely to develop greenstick type fractures with entrapment of extraoccular musculature and other soft tissue.

PRESENTATION OF FRACTURES

Mandible

The incidence of pediatric facial fractures had been estimated at 1 to 15 % of all facial fractures including adults and children[10] Mandibular fractures represent approximately 15 to 20% of pediatric facial fractures.[10] Some of the more

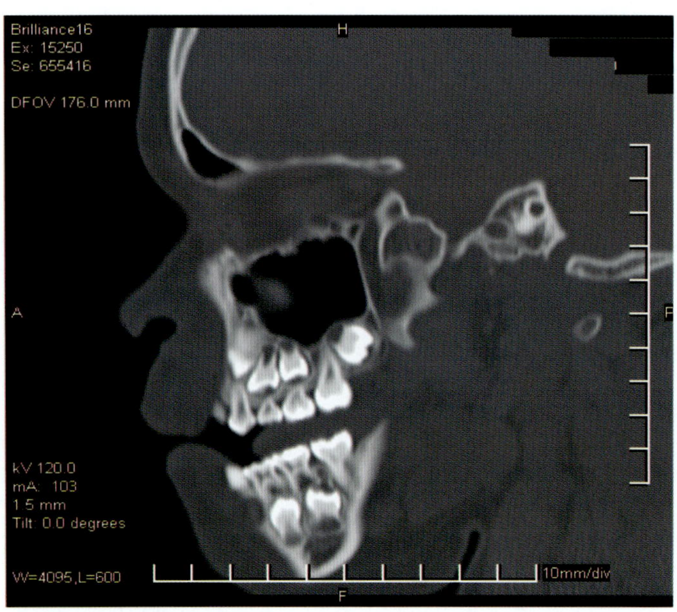

Fig 8–1. Unerupted pediatric teeth.

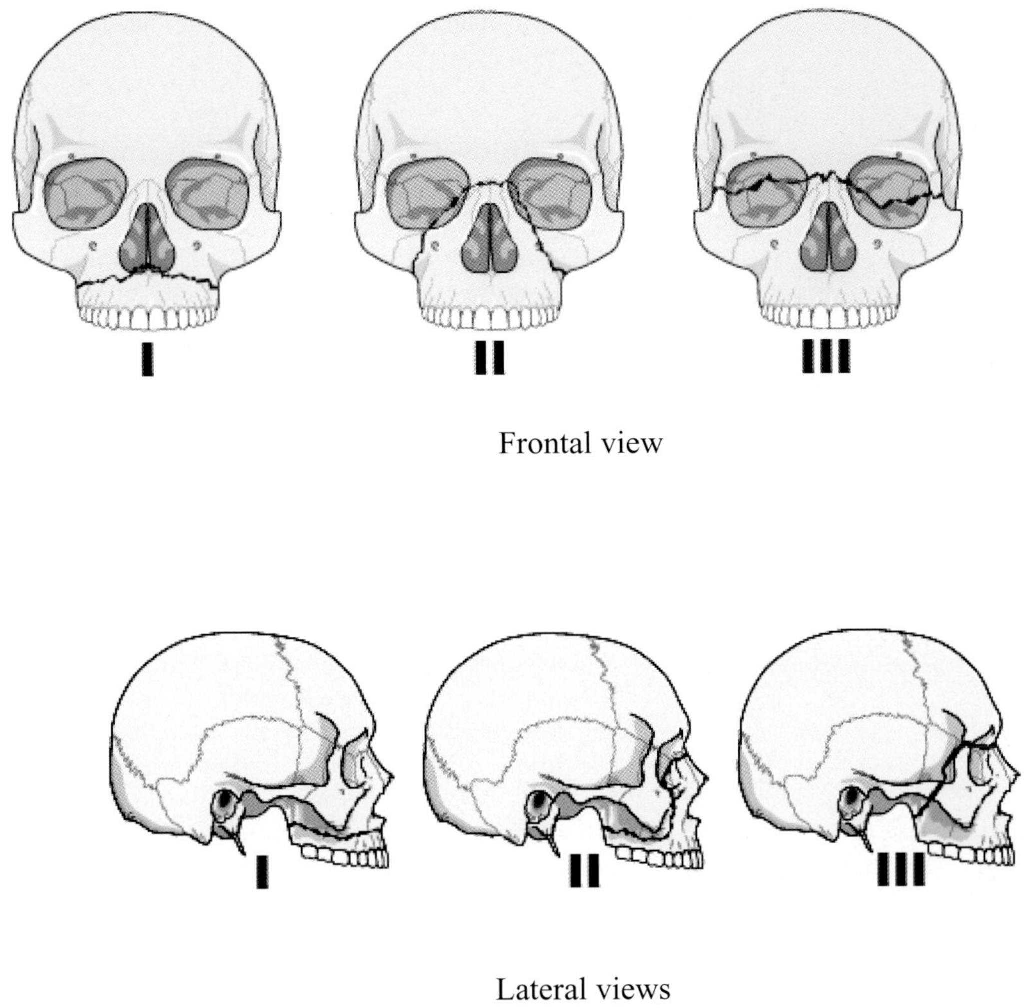

Fig 8–2. Le Fort fractures I, II, and III with frontal and lateral view.

common mechanisms were covered previously. They include motor vehicle collision, falls, and sports-related injuries in decreasing order. Because mandible fractures are more commonly seen in high-velocity incidents, it is common to see accompanying injuries to the neurocranium, and orthopedic and intra-abdominal injuries.[10,11]

Condylar fractures can be divided into three types: comminuted, high, and low. Comminuted and high condylar fractures are considered intracapusular. Low condylar fractures are considered extracapsular. The most common condylar fracture is the low subcondylar fracture that occurs below the sigmoid notch (Fig 8–3). It is important to realize that, as the condylar head develops, growth is downward toward the angle. Because of this, the condylar neck begins as a short, thick segment that then elongates. This is why whereas low subcondylar fractures are most common overall, crush injures involving the articular surface are the most common fractures in children less than 5 years old. Clear knowledge of the anatomy of the temporal mandibular joint is key to the understanding of the presentation and complication. Some of the more common presentations of condylar fractures are the inability to open the mouth, echymosis and pain over the temporal mandibular joint, and echymosis and edema of the posterior external auditory canal. Important complications involve facial asymmetry, repair complications such as infection and hardware extrusions, VII cranial nerve palsy, displacement of the fracture segments into the middle cranial fossa, and hemarthrosis due to the high vascularity of the condyle. There is debate over the risk for ankylosis with hemarthrosis.[12,13] The more common complication of condylar fracture is disruption in growth patterns. It is

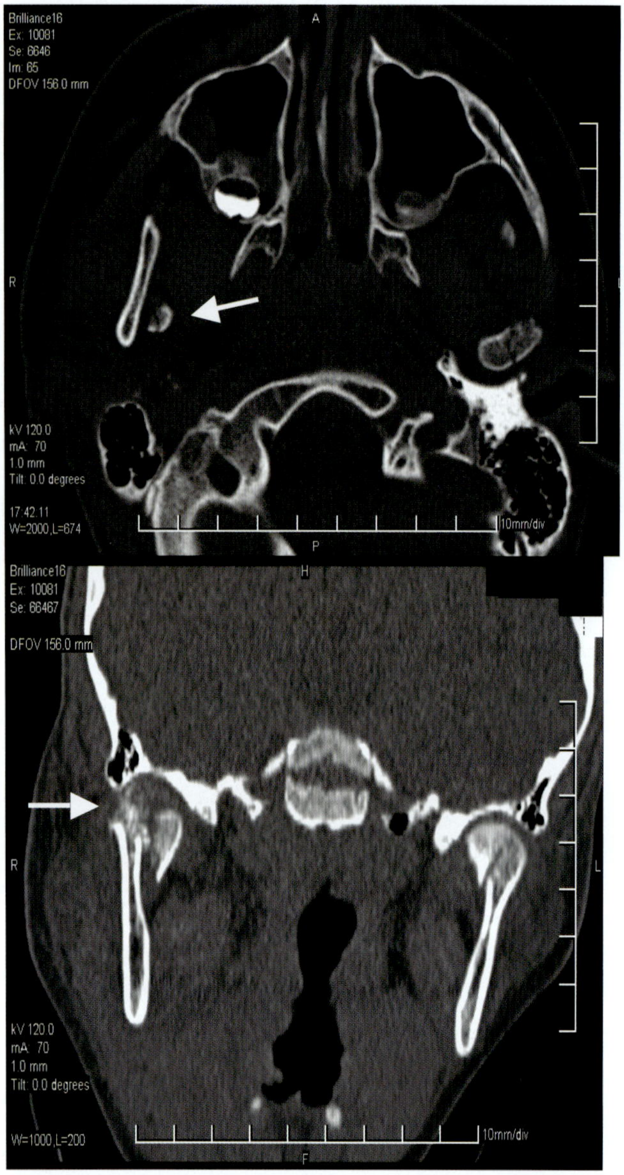

Fig 8–3. Mandibular condyle and subcondylar fracture. Child involved in MVC. Reconstructed coronal image below demonstrates the comminuted, impacted, and displaced fracture of the right mandibular condyle. The loss of the normal articulation with the glenoid fossa is revealed on both axial and coronal images.

recognized that the condyle is an important growth center. Also, the level of remolding in this area decreases with age. These factors have been used to explain why younger children who suffer from condylar fractures have decreased long-term morbidity.[11,14]

Arch, Body, Symphaseal, Parasymphaseal, and Dentoalveolar

The mandibular arch, body, symphaseal, parasymphaseal, and dentoalveolar fracture sites have similar presentations and complications. Commonly these fractures cause asymmetric change in the mandible, tooth damage, alteration in the function of attached musculature, and damage to surrounding neurovascular bundles. Beginning with neurovascular bundle damage, on the buccal surface of the mandible courses the inferior alveolar nerve and vasculature. It extends to exit the mandible at the mental foramen. Disruption can lead to parasthesia, anesthesia, and bleeding. In addition, the action of the muscular pull and masticatory forces frequently dislocate bony segments making it necessary to perform rigid fixation. Dentoalveolar and body fractures usually involve tooth damage. Placement of primary teeth does not improve outcome unless used to maintain dental alignment until permanent dentition erupts. In contrast, permanent teeth should be replaced within 2 hours of injury. If unable to be replaced before evaluation by a medical professional, transport should be done in saline type solution or milk.

Orbital

Orbital fractures among children are uncommon. This is again related to the anatomy of the child face in relationship to the skull.[15] When orbital fractures occur the most common cause is sport or play related. Although children have an increased amount of cancellous cortical bone, which provides some flexibility in the facial structure compared to adults, it requires a significant amount of force to cause orbital fractures. This is why there is an increased risk of associated injuries in orbital fractures compared to other pediatric facial fractures. Hatton et al found that 50% of child orbital fractures had associated intraocular injury.[16] Intracranial injuries can also occur. There are several types of orbital fractures. To address specific complication and related injuries it is best to divide orbital fractures into fracture units. The most common fracture of the orbit involves the lateral orbit and zygoma. These injuries can involve damage to the lateral canthal ligament and or entrapment of the lateral rectus. This presents as lower lid ptosis and restricted extraoccular movement, respectively. Medial orbital fractures frequently result in disruption of the medial collateral ligament and the lacrimal duct system. Orbital zygomatic fractures are commonly seen with orbital floor fractures (Fig 8–4). Although commonly involved with orbital fractures, zygoma fractures can also occur alone (Fig 8–5). A second anatomic fact to highlight is that facial fractures, particularly orbital, are influenced by development of the paranasal sinuses. At birth the maxillary sinus is medial to the orbit. By age 7 the maxillary sinus expands laterally. Also, the ethmoid sinuses are 70% developed by this point. Because of this development, orbital floor fractures are uncommon before the age of 5 years old.[1] The adult orbital floor is thin and rigid which results in comminuted fractures. Comparatively, the pediatric orbital floor is flexible and produces "trap-door" fractures with associated entrapment of the inferior rectus (Fig 8–6). Entrapment of the inferior rectus or periorbital fat is associated with nausea and vomiting from edema caused by increased intraorbital pressure or necroses of entrapped tissue.[17] Other symptoms commonly seen in orbital floor fractures are parasthesia or anesthesia over the anterior cheek, upper lip, and maxillary gingiva secondary to inferior orbital nerve damage.

Just as maxillary and ethmoid sinus development influence orbital floor and medial orbital fractures, frontal sinus development influences the potential of superior orbital wall fractures. In the adult, the frontal sinus helps dissipate impact energy and provide some protection from orbital roof fracture. The development of sinuses and the increased ratio of cranium to midface result in increased superior orbital wall fractures in children compared to

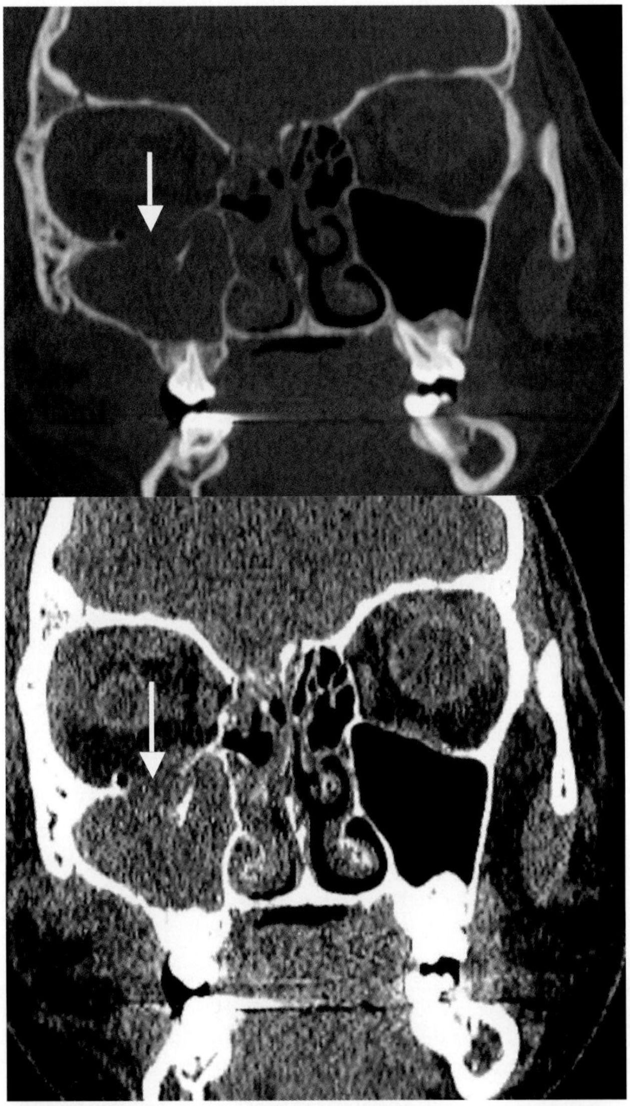

Fig 8–4. Orbital fracture. As with orbital floor fractures, these axial plane fractures are often best displayed in the coronal or sagittal plane. The two images provided are at the same location: above, displayed at bone window and level settings; below, displayed at soft tissue window and level settings.

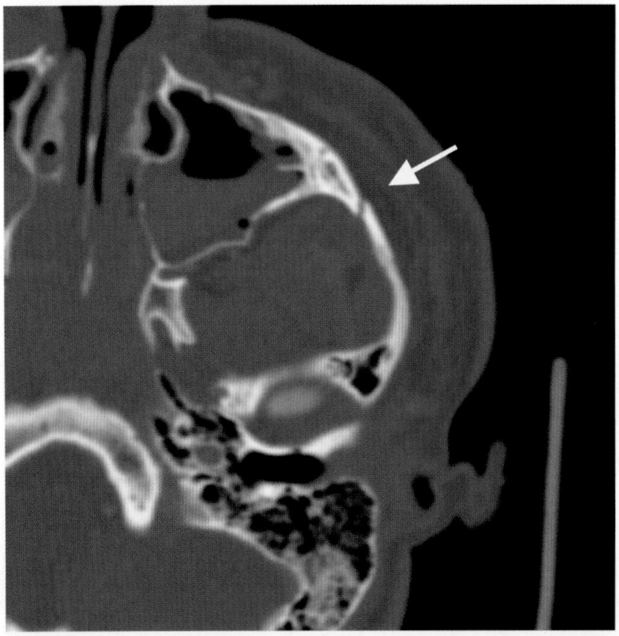

Fig 8–5. Isolated zygoma fracture.

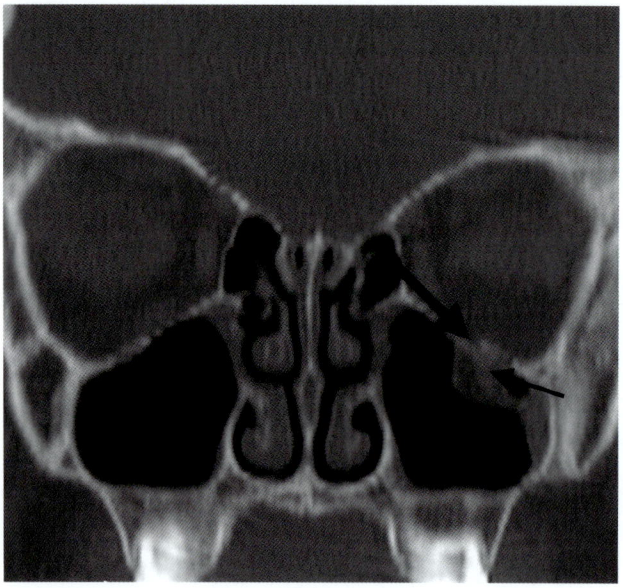

Fig 8–6. "Trap-door" fracture with inferior rectus entrapped (*thin arrow*). Note that the fracture is not depressed. (*thick arrow*).

adults. Orbital roof fractures do not usually result in entrapment but do commonly involve the supraorbital and supratrochlear neurovascular complex leading to altered sensation to corresponding areas. In the evaluation of children with orbital fractures it is important to involve ophthalmology. This is required because of possible ruptured globe, orbital hematoma, optic nerve sheath hematoma, and/or retinal detachment.[18] The most common orbital fracture resulting in blindness is an orbital apex fracture. These fractures result from high-energy injuries and are frequently observed post mortem. Rarely is there complete resolution of the visual defects.

Nose

Nasal fractures are the most common pediatric facial fracture. As discussed earlier, they commonly result from falls, motor vehicle collisions, or sports.[19] The nasal framework includes both bony and cartilaginous portion. The nasal bones are paired and fuse with the frontal bone superiorly and the maxilla laterally. It is supported medially by the septum. Cartilaginous structures include the paired upper lateral cartilages, which extend beneath the nasal bones, and the lower lateral nasal cartilages. Nasal trauma can obviously lead to cosmetic issues; however, there can also be more serious complications to include long-term nasal functional defects, septal hematoma, septal abscess, lacrimal duct obstruction, alteration in facial growth, and or naso-oral fistulas (Fig 8–7).

Nasal hematomas and abscesses are related in their etiology. The nasal cavity has a rich blood supply from both the internal and external carotid. Trauma that results in disruption of the cartilage and overlying mucoperichondrium can lead to hematoma formation. This causes necrosis of the septum by both pressure necrosis and avascular necrosis. The latter occurs because the mucoperichondrium is the nutrient source for the underlying cartilage. Infection can closely follow hematoma formation and necrosis leading to septal abscess.[20,21] Infection usually involves nasal flora and requires broad-spectrum antibiotics and drainage. Both septal abscess and hematoma are a surgical emergency because they can lead to septal perforation, facial deformity, and nasal malfunction.[22] Nasal oral fistulas are a rare complication and there has been one case report.[23] Ousterhout observed that midface fractures including a nasal septal fracture which could lead to midface retrusion needed iatrogenic Le Fort type III fracture to repair.[24]

Other Complications

Although the temporal bone is not considered part of the facial skeleton, fractures of the temporal bone can be seen with facial fractures. In fact 30 to 70% of blunt head trauma has a temporal bone component.[25] There are three types of temporal bone fractures: longitudinal, transverse, and combined. Longitudinal fractures are the most common. These fractures extend in a plane parallel to the facial nerve. Transverse temporal fractures on the other hand extend to transect the facial nerve. Complications of temporal bone fractures include hearing loss from damage to inner or middle ear components or to the vestibulocochlear nerve and facial nerve damage. Hearing loss is seen in 37 to 81% of pediatric temporal bone fractures. Cerebrospinal fluid leak is another complication of temporal bone fractures, and occurs in up to 25%. It is important to follow children with temporal bone fractures as outpatients because there have been reports of delayed onset of cranial nerve deficits.[25,26]

Facial nerve damage is possible with any of the facial skeletal trauma discussed above. Three percent of pediatric

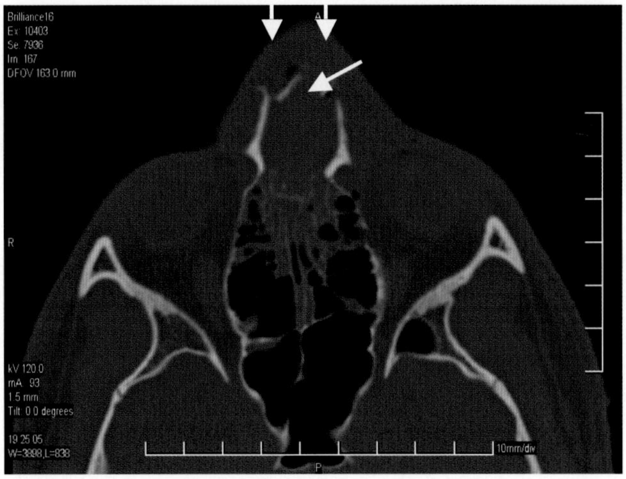

Fig 8–7. Bilateral nasal bone fractures.

temporal bone fractures cause facial paralysis. Management of the paralysis depends on presentation and electoneurography. It has been found that surgical exploration with decompression and/or reanastomosis is best with complete paralysis on presentation with greater than 95% degeneration on electroneurography. This decision must be made within the first 14 days. If either the presentation, degeneration, or time between onset and management dose not meet this criteria, observation with later surgical management as needed is advised.[25,27] With any laceration or injury to the midface, injury to the parotid duct should also be considered. The parotid duct travels across the midface with the buccal branch of the facial nerve. Damage to the parotid duct should be repaired and the facial nerve should also be evaluated and followed for delayed paralysis. Failure to repair the parotid can lead to sialoadenitis or sialocele formation.

CONCLUSION

Pediatric facial fractures are complicated injuries that require a diverse team of physicians to adequately care for the injuries. Imaging is critical for management planning. Plans for repair should consider bony growth dynamics as iatrogenic disruption of soft tissue and bony structures can alter growth. The pediatric face is developing and thus these dynamic changes lead to alterations in patterns of fractures as the face matures. It is important to evaluate children thoroughly for the complications discussed to minimize the morbidity of facial fractures.

REFERENCES

1. Cummings CW. *Otolaryngolgy: Head and Neck Surgery.* 4th ed. St. Louis, Mo: Mosby; 2005.
2. Langlois JA. *Traumatic Brain Injury in the United States: Assessing Outcomes in Children.* Atlanta, Ga: National Center for Injury Prevention and Control, Centers for Disease Control and Prevention (CDC); 2001.
3. Children's Safety Network Economics and Insurance Resource Center Data and Surveillance. *Economic Cost and Comparison of Injury.* Fact sheet packet. 1966.
4. Enlow DH. *Facial Growth.* 3rd ed. Philadelphia, Pa: WB Saunders; 1990.
5. Chan J. The age-dependent relationship between facial fractures and skull fractures. *Int J Ped Otorhinolaryngol.* 2004;68:877–881.
6. Seiden A. *Otolaryngology: The Essentials.* New York, NY: Thieme; 2002:77–84.
7. Cawood JL. Facial trauma. *Int J Oral Maxillofac Surg.* 1990;19:193.
8. Oji C. Fractures of the facial skeleton in children: a survey of patients under the age of 11 years. *J Craniomoxillofac Surg.* 1998;26(5):322–325.
9. Iizuka T. Midfacial fractures in pediatric patients. Frequency, characteristics and causes. *Arch Otolaryngol Head Neck Surg.* 1995;121(12):1366–1371.
10. Smartt J. The pediatric mandible. II Management of traumatic injury or fracture. *Plast Reconstr Surg.* 2005; 116(2):28e–41e.
11. Schweinfurth J. Pediatric mandibular fractures. *Facial Plast Surg.* 1998;14:31–44.
12. Oztan HY. The role of trauma on temporomandibular joint ankylosis and mandibular growth retardation: an experimental study. *J Craniofac Surg.* 2004;14(2):274–282.
13. Ferreira P. Etiology and patterns of pediatric mandibular fractures in Portugal: a retrospective study of 10 years. *J Craniofac Surg.* 2004;15(3):384–391.
14. Norholt S. Pediatric condylar fractures: in a long-term follow-up study of 55 patients. *J Craniomaxillofac Surg.* 1993;51:1302–1310.
15. Neuman MI. *Textbook of Pediatric Emergency Medicine.* 5th ed. Fleisher GLS, Henretig, R, eds. Philadelphia, Pa: Lippincott Williams & Wilkins; 2005:1475.
16. Hatton, MP. Orbital fractures in children. *Ophthal Plast Reconstr Surg.* 2001;17:174–179.

17. Jatia KK. Orbital fractures: a review of current literature. *Curr Surg.* 2004;61:25–29.
18. Long J. Orbital trauma. *Ophthalmol Clin North Am.* 2002; 15:249–253.
19. Anderson PJ. *Fractures of the facial skeleton in children. Injury.* 1995;26:47–50.
20. Olsen KD. Nasal septal injury in children. Diagnosis and management. *Arch Otolaryngol.* 1980;106:317–320.
21. Ginsburg CM. Infected nasal septal hematoma. *Ped Infect Dis J.* 1995;14:1012–1013.
22. Grymer LF. The nasal septum and the development of the midface. A longitudinal study of a pair of monozygotic twins. *Rhinology.* 1997;35:6–10.
23. Cuddihy PJ. An unusual presentation of a nasal septal abscess. *J Laryngol Otol.* 1998;112(8):775–776.
24. Ousterhout DK. Maxillary hypoplasia secondary to midfacial trauma in childhood. *Plast Reconstr Surg.* 1987; 80(4):491–499.
25. Yildirim A. Fracture of the skull base with delayed multiple cranial nerve palsies. *Ped Emerg Care.* 2005;21(7): 440–442.
26. Lee D. Pediatric temporal bone fractures. *Laryngoscope.* 1998;108(6):816–820.
27. Chang C. Management of facial nerve injury due to temporal bone trauma. *Am J Otol.* 1999;20:96–114.

9

Imaging of Pediatric Facial Fractures

Amanda Corey

The mainstay of current imaging to evaluate facial trauma and confirm the clinical suspicion of facial fracture is CT. High-resolution, thin-section, axial image acquisition is performed. The image data can then be manipulated and displayed using either the Picture Archives Communications System (PACS) work station or a separate vendor work station for viewing the images in the desired fashion (eg, axial or coronal plane, soft tissue or bone window/level, 3-dimensional display), thus providing versatility and excellent anatomic detail.

When reviewing at the PACS station, the images can be evaluated at various window and level settings to optimize demonstration of soft tissues or osseous structures (Fig 9–1). Multiplanar reconstructions are particularly useful in the evaluation of anatomic structures in the axial plane such as the orbital floor and roof, the hard palate, and the

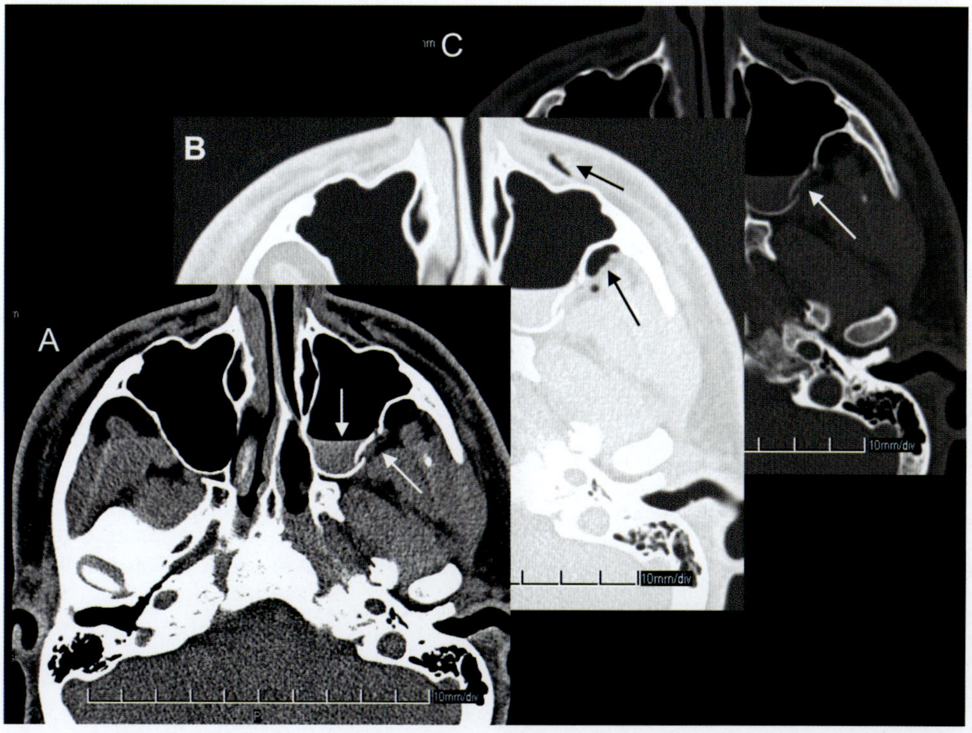

Fig 9–1. Different tissue technique displays. Axial CT images from an 8-year-old child following a fall from a bicycle. Image A is displayed at "Soft tissue" technique. The left maxillary sinus air-fluid level and the hematoma in the retroantral location are well seen. Image B is displayed at "Lung" technique. The air in the premalar soft tissue and in the retroantral location are easily noted. Image C is displayed at "Bone" technique. The minimally displayed lateral maxillary sinus wall fracture is visible.

craniocervical junction. Osseous derangement superiorly-inferiorly, left-right, or anterior-posterior can be confirmed and sometimes better demonstrated on coronal and sagittal reformations than on the axial image (Fig 9–2).

CT evaluation of the face includes assessment for:

- Soft tissue asymmetry of edema or hematoma
- Foreign bodies
- Air, fat, soft tissue, or bone where it does not belong
- Bone contour abnormality of greenstick fracture or frank "step-off" of displaced fractures
- Associated injuries.

Superficial hematomas or areas of soft tissue injury as indicated by skin avulsion, soft tissue swelling, and subcutaneous fat stranding can provide a radiographic clue to look more closely in that area for underlying fracture (Figs 9–3 and 9–4).

A normal tissue in an abnormal location (orbital fat or the inferior rectus muscle prolapsing into the maxillary sinus, for example) should prompt assessment for underlying fracture. In Figure 9–5, the mandibular condyle has been displaced through the roof of the condylar fossa and into the temporal lobe of the brain. Orbital emphysema occurs with penetrating trauma, or, more commonly, when fractures create a communication with an adjacent pneumatized paranasal sinus (Fig 9–6). Blood or blood/fluid and air levels in a paranasal sinus are another clue to fracture involving that sinus. As shown in Figure 9-1, air and hematoma in the retroantral fat are abnormal findings and can be seen in association with fractures of the posterior-lateral wall of the maxillary sinus.

Sometimes fractures are subtle, with loss of normal contour to the osseous structure. In those cases, comparison with the unaffected side is useful in making the diagnosis (Fig 9–7). In other instances, fractures present as obvious discontinuity, displacement, distraction, or angulation of the affected bone (Fig 9–8).

In the general assessment of a child with facial trauma, associated injuries should be sought as they are found in 25 to 75% of patients. The incidence of associated injury increases with the severity of the identified trauma. Thus, patients with midface fractures and severely displaced fractures are at increased risk for injuries to the spine, brain,

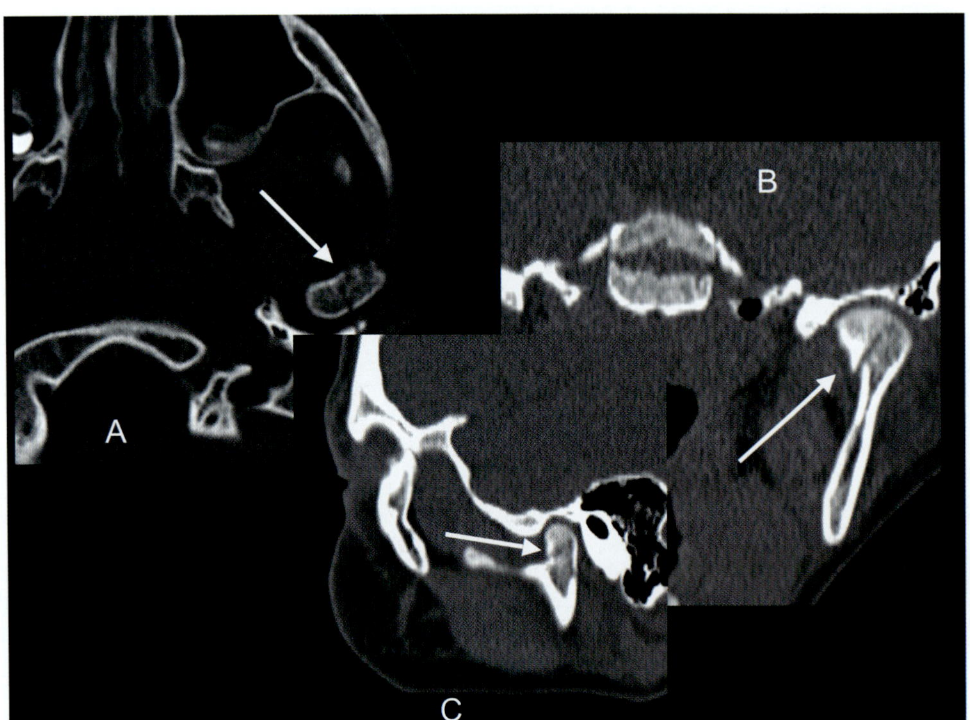

Fig 9–2. Multiplanar display. Left mandibular condylar head fracture displayed in the axial (A), coronal (B), and sagittal (C) planes. Although the fracture is intra-articular and there is slight displacement in the transverse plane (shown in B); the condyle is not displaced from the articular fossa.

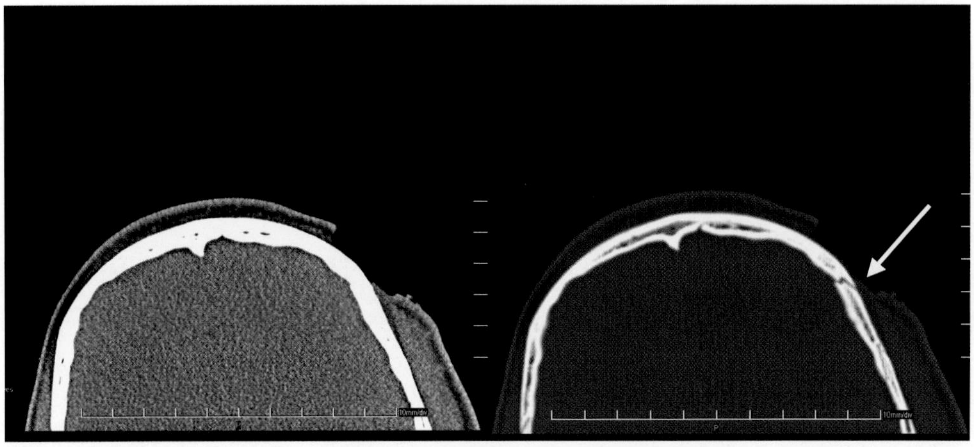

Fig 9–3. Scalp avulsion. Axial CT images obtained above the orbits demonstrates a full-thickness avulsion injury with a scalp defect on the left. The arrow in the second image (displayed at bone window and level setting) reveals the underlying nondisplaced calvarial fracture.

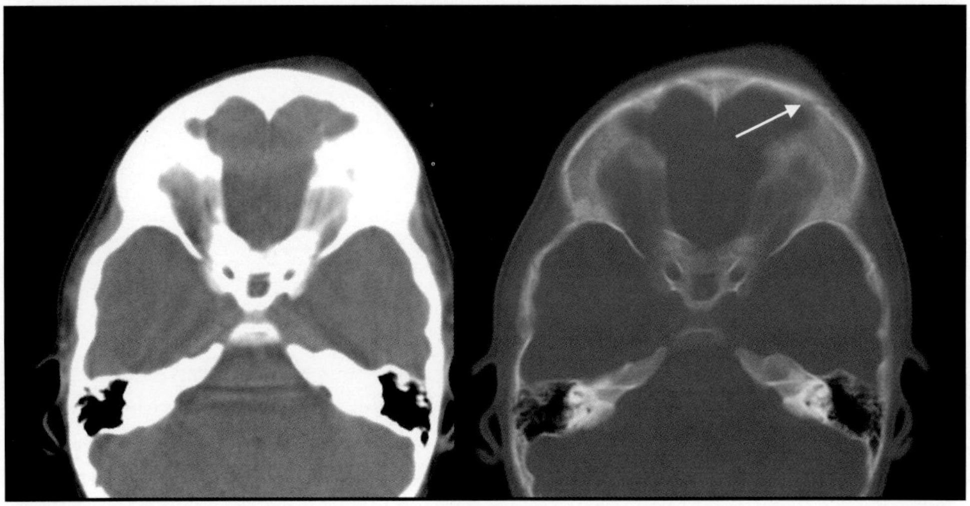

Fig 9–4. Scalp hematoma. This 4-year-old male presented to the emergency room following a fall. The image on the left shows the left supraorbital scalp hematoma. The image on the right includes a portion of the nondisplaced frontal bone fracture (arrow). Noncontrast head CT should also be obtained to assess for the full fracture extent as well as any associated injuries such as extra-axial blood or parenchymal contusions.

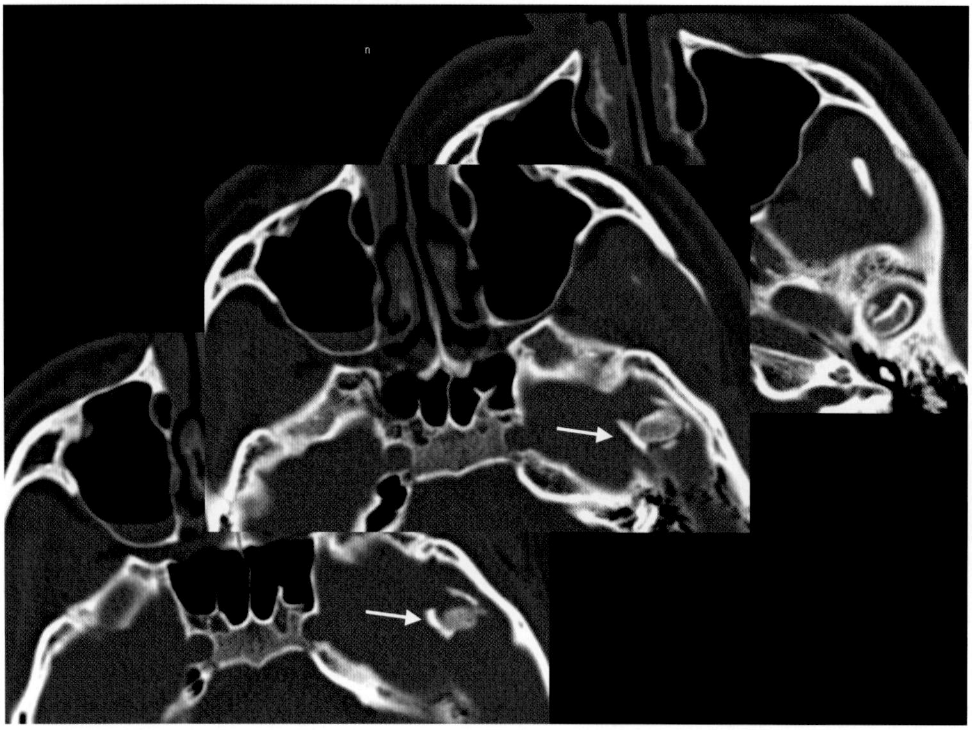

Fig 9–5. Displaced mandibular condyle fracture. The left mandibular condyle has been displaced through the condylar fossa, into the middle cranial fossa and temporal lobe of the brain.

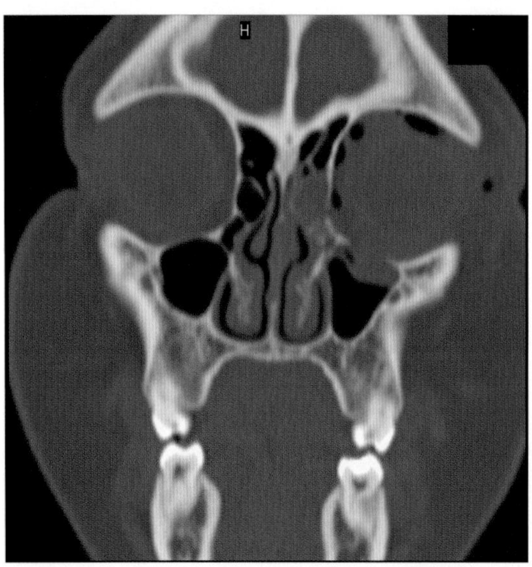

Fig 9–6. Orbital blow-out fractures with orbital emphysema. Orbital emphysema is noted in association with a fracture of the left orbital floor and the left lamina papyracea. Blood is seen in the adjacent left ethmoid air cells. Orbital contents and hemorrhage are seen prolapsing into the maxillary sinus.

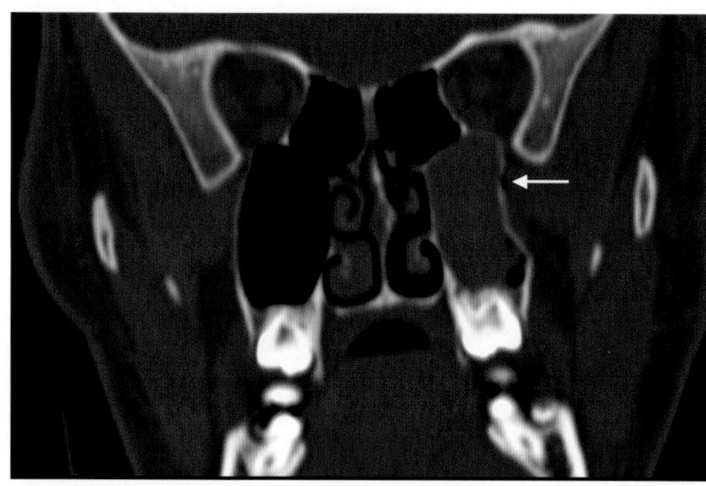

Fig 9–7. Sinus wall fracture. This 10-year-old patient was involved in bicycle versus automobile accident. The lateral wall of the left maxillary sinus has lost the regular, slightly convex and smooth contour shown on the right. Fluid/blood is present in the left maxillary sinus and a tiny focus of air (*arrow*) is noted outside the sinus, within the adjacent soft tissues, in this pediatric patient with a minimally displaced sinus wall fracture.

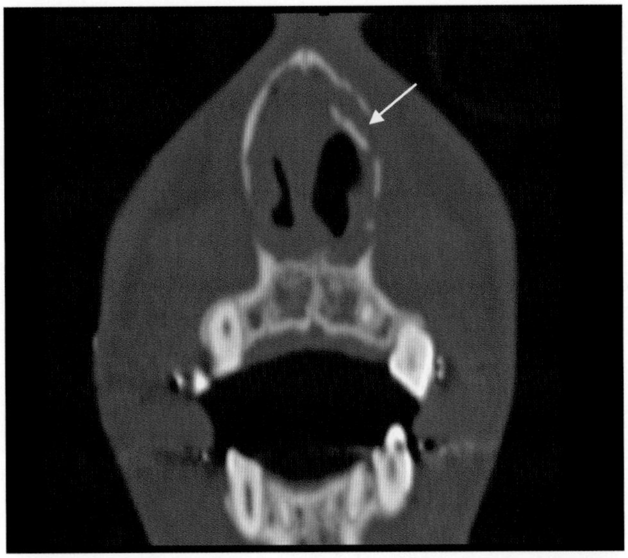

Fig 9–8. Nasal bone fracture. This middle school student came to the Emergency Room after a fight at school. The coronal reconstructed image shows a displaced and comminuted fracture of the left nasal bone.

torso, or extremities as compared with patients who have suffered a lower impact injury[1] (Figs 9–9 through 9–14).

As stated elsewhere in this text, the pattern and location of fractures in children not only varies with the mechanism and velocity of injury, but also with the age of the patient. Facial development, flexibility of the skeleton, and likelihood of exposure to trauma all factor into the injury patterns of children.[2]

Dentoalveolar and nasal fractures are common pediatric facial fractures. However, many of these injuries do not present to the radiologist for diagnosis by CT imaging (Fig 9–15).When a fracture of the nasal bones, palate, or frontal process of the maxilla is found, assessment of the septum for hematoma should be performed

After nasal bone fractures, mandibular fractures are the second-most common facial fracture in children.[1] Mandibular condylar fractures are the most common mandibular fractures in children and are more commonly seen in children than in adults. In children under 6, intracapsular fractures are more likely. In children over 6, fractures are more likely to occur in the neck of the mandible. In

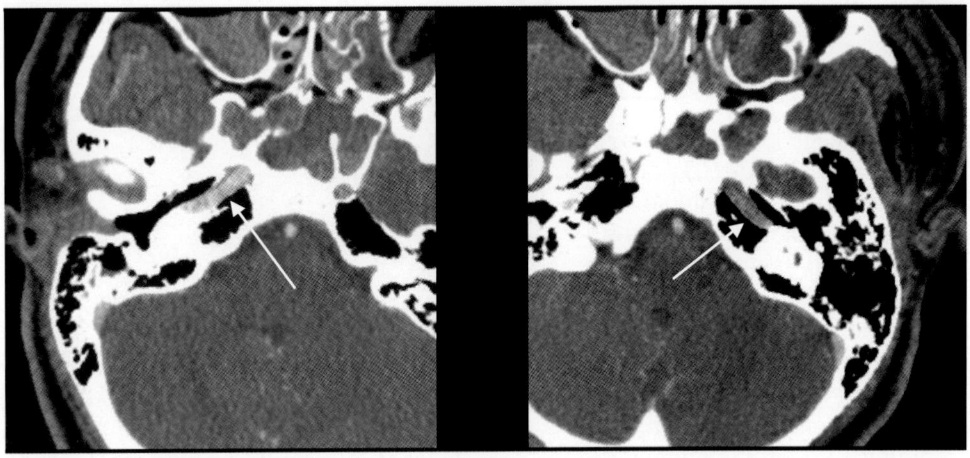

Fig 9–9. Carotid occlusion. This 13-year-old patient was involved in a high-speed motor vehicle collision. Initial facial CT revealed facial and skull base fractures including a fracture of the sphenoid bone in the region of the carotid canal. CTA was then performed to assess the integrity of the internal carotid artery. The figure on the left shows intravascular contrast in the patent horizontal petrous segment of the ICA. The figure on the right shows lack of intravascular contrast in the left horizontal petrous segment of the ICA. Traumatic dissection and occlusion of the left ICA is proved. Blood products (high-density material) in the paranasal sinuses is also present. In the figure on the left, the lateral and septal wall fracture of the right sphenoid chamber can be seen.

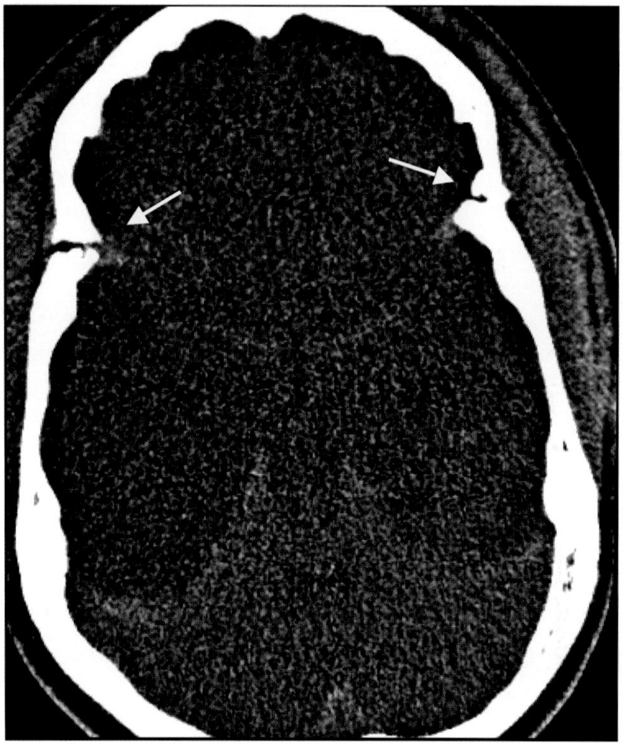

Fig 9–10. Profound hypoxic ischemic injury in the setting of trauma. This 8-year-old patient was ejected from a car suffering multiple internal injuries and reportedly arrested at the scene. Massive brain swelling is present with effacement of the basilar cisterns. The gray matter—white matter distinction is lost in the supratentorial brain giving the brain parenchyma a bland low attenuation. The "dense cerebellar" sign of relative sparing of the brainstem and cerebellum is due in part to autoregulation variation between the anterior and posterior circulation and demand differences. Bilateral anterior calvarial fracture lines are visible at the level of the pterion (*arrows*).

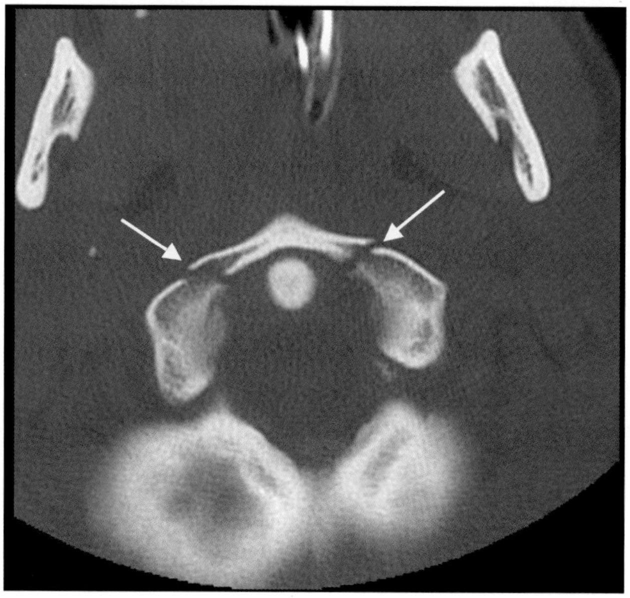

Fig 9–11. Cervical spine fracture. 16-year-old involved in a high-speed MVA. The anterior arch of C1 ring has fractured in two places (arrows). The patient had severely depressed frontal bone fractures in addition.

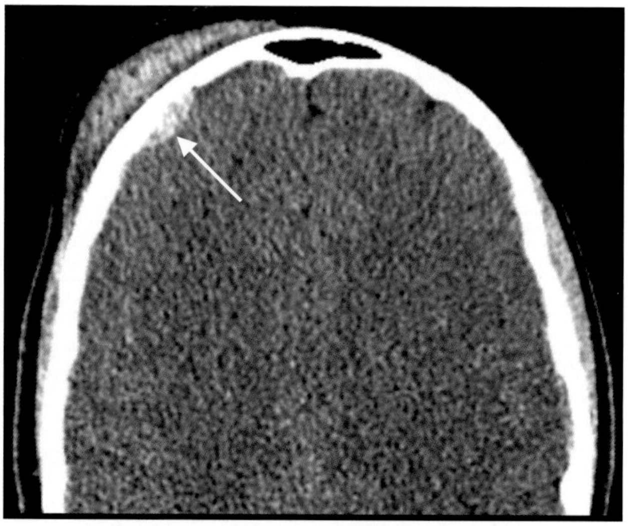

Fig 9–12. Extra-axial hematoma (*arrow*) beneath sentinel scalp hematoma.

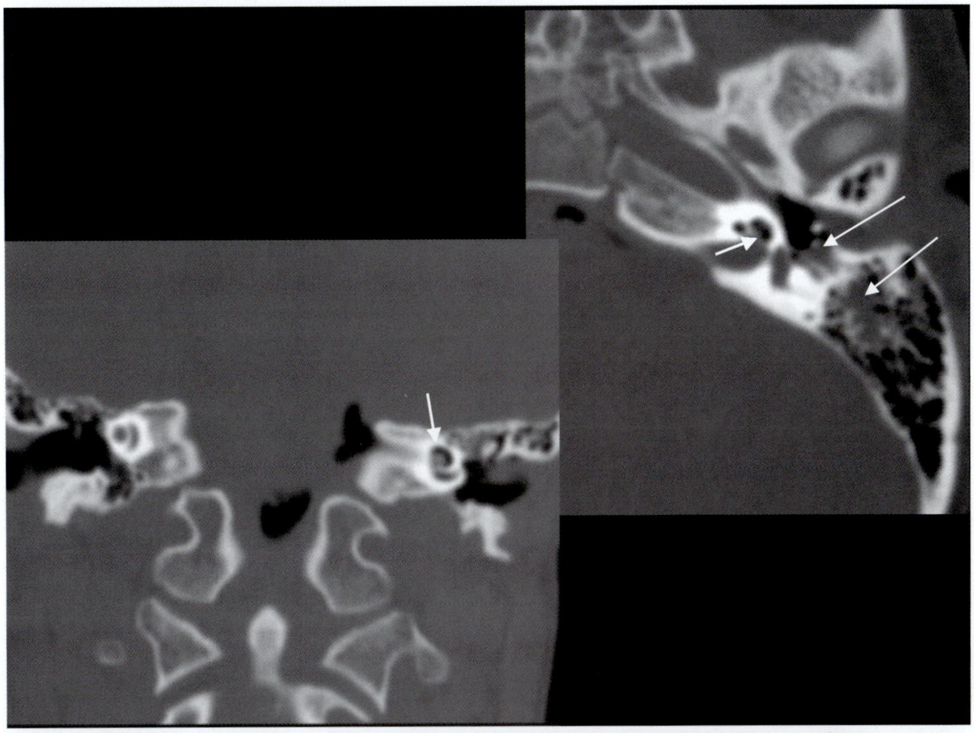

Fig 9–13. Pneumolabyrinth. Image on the left is a coronal reformat at the level of the cochlea. Image on the right is in the axial orientation at the level of the internal auditory canal. Air is present in the left cochlea (*short arrow on both images*) and intracranially. The middle ear and mastoid air cells are partly opacified (*long arrows*). Underlying temporal bone fracture should be sought.

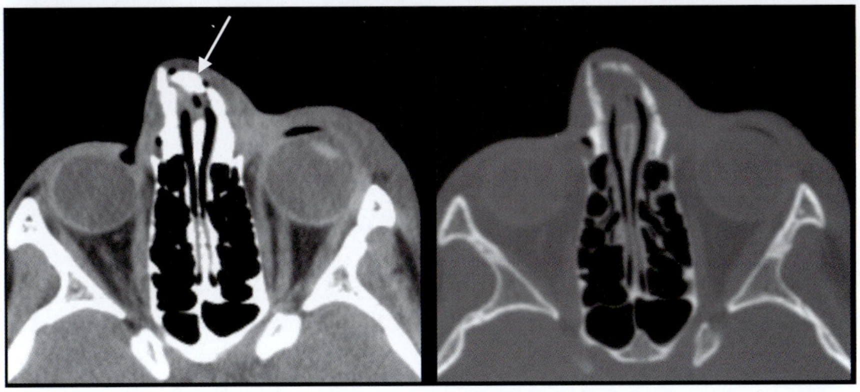

Fig 9–14. Bilateral nasal bone fractures with depression of the central fragment (*arrow*). Injury was sustained in a MVC.

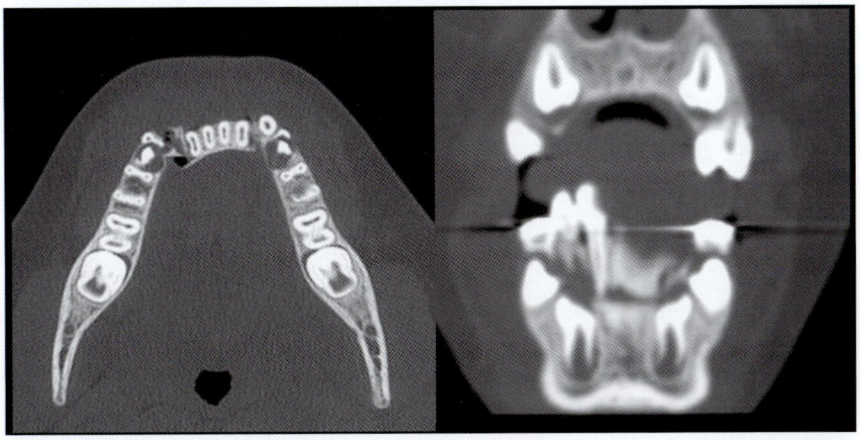

Fig 9–15. Segmental alveolar fracture. Axial image on the left (*bone algorithm*) and coronal reformat (*soft tissue alogrithm displayed at bone window and level setting*) image on the right demonstrate the displaced and diastatic fracture of the parasymphyseal mandibular alveolar ridge. In this 9-year-old boy, notice the mixture of primary and permanent dentition. The coronal reconstruction helps demonstrate the relationship of the teeth to the fracture line.

decreasing order of incidence, other fractures of the mandible in children include those affecting the symphysis, angle, and body (Figs 9–16 through 9–20).[2]

Orbital fractures are seen with increasing frequency as pneumatization of the paranasal sinuses proceeds. When assessing the orbit, attention should be paid to the inferior orbital nerve canal, the integrity of the globe and orbital contents, and findings to suggest blood products in the intraconal, extraconal, or intramuscular locations. Entrapment of the extraocular muscles is often suspected

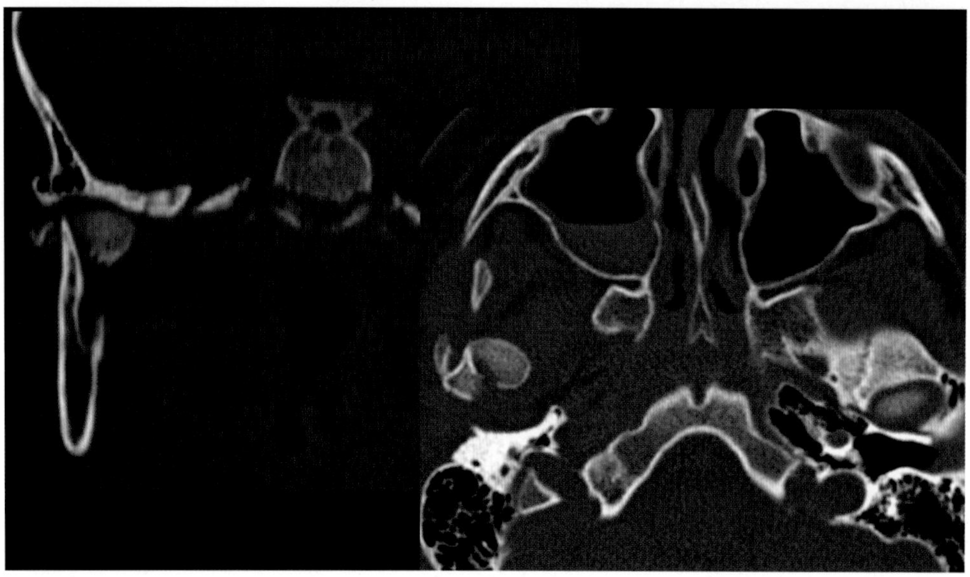

Fig 9–16. Mandibular condyle and subcondylar fracture. 10-year-old child involved in MVC. Reconstructed coronal image on the left and axial image on the right demonstrate the comminuted, impacted, and displaced fracture of the right mandibular condyle. The loss of the normal articulation with the glenoid fossa is revealed on both axial and coronal images.

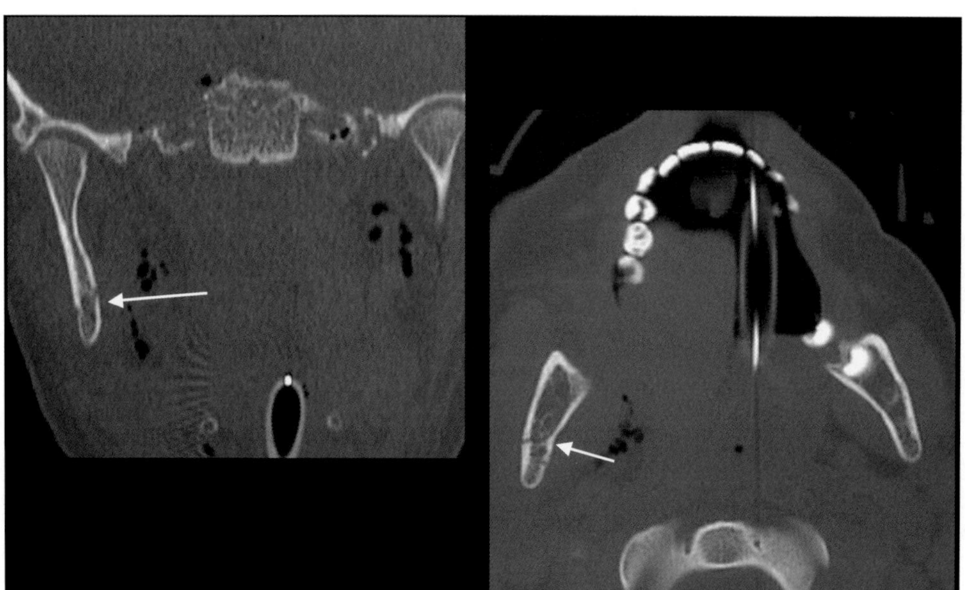

Fig 9–17. Fracture of the mandibular angle. This 11-year-old was involved in a MVC. A nondisplaced fracture through the right mandibular angle involves the canal for the inferior alveolar nerve, as demonstrated on the coronal reconstructed image (bone algorithm). On the axial image presented, the fracture line passes posterior to the canal. Note the endotracheal tube on the axial image. Air in the parapharyngeal spaces bilaterally raises the question of a mucosal injury.

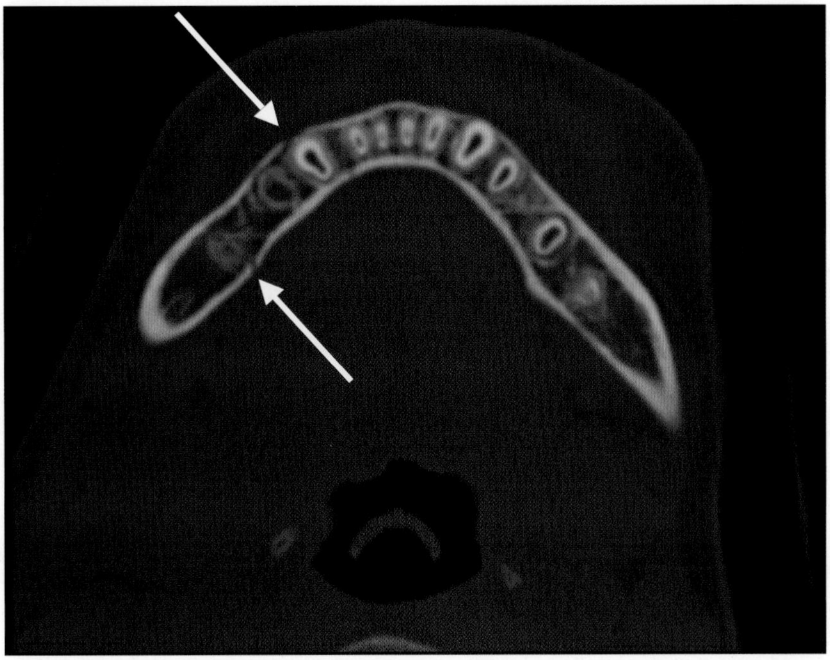

Fig 9–18. Mandibular body fracture. This 10-year-old MVA victim has a nondisplaced fracture of the mid and anterior right mandibular body extending beyond the mental foramen and into the parasymphaseal region of the mandible. The fracture line is subtle, but the loss of cortical continuity can be seen on both the lingual and buccal surface of the mandible.

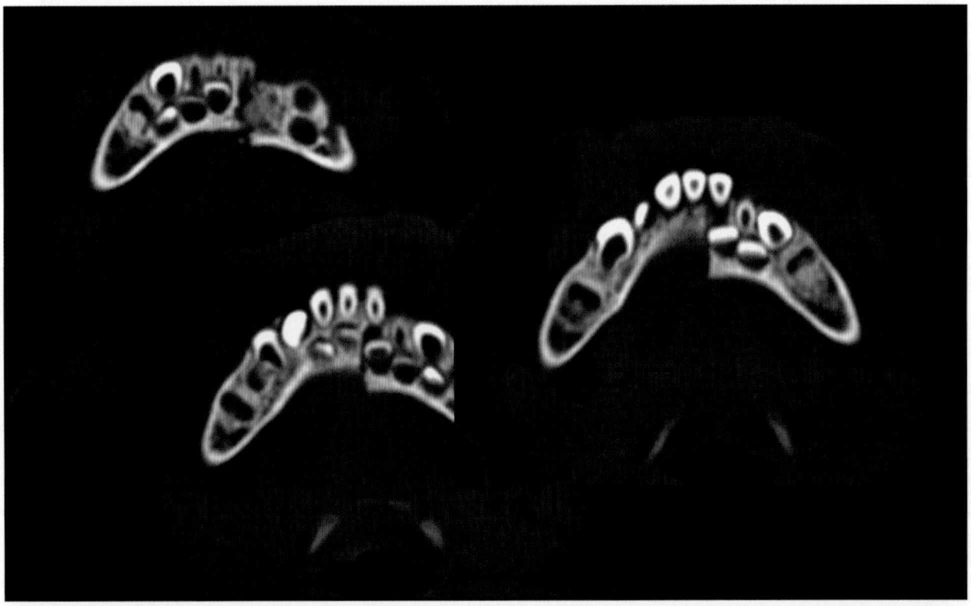

Fig 9–19. Parasymphyseal mandibular fracture. Posterior displacement of the left hemi-mandible relative to the right is noted on the axial images.

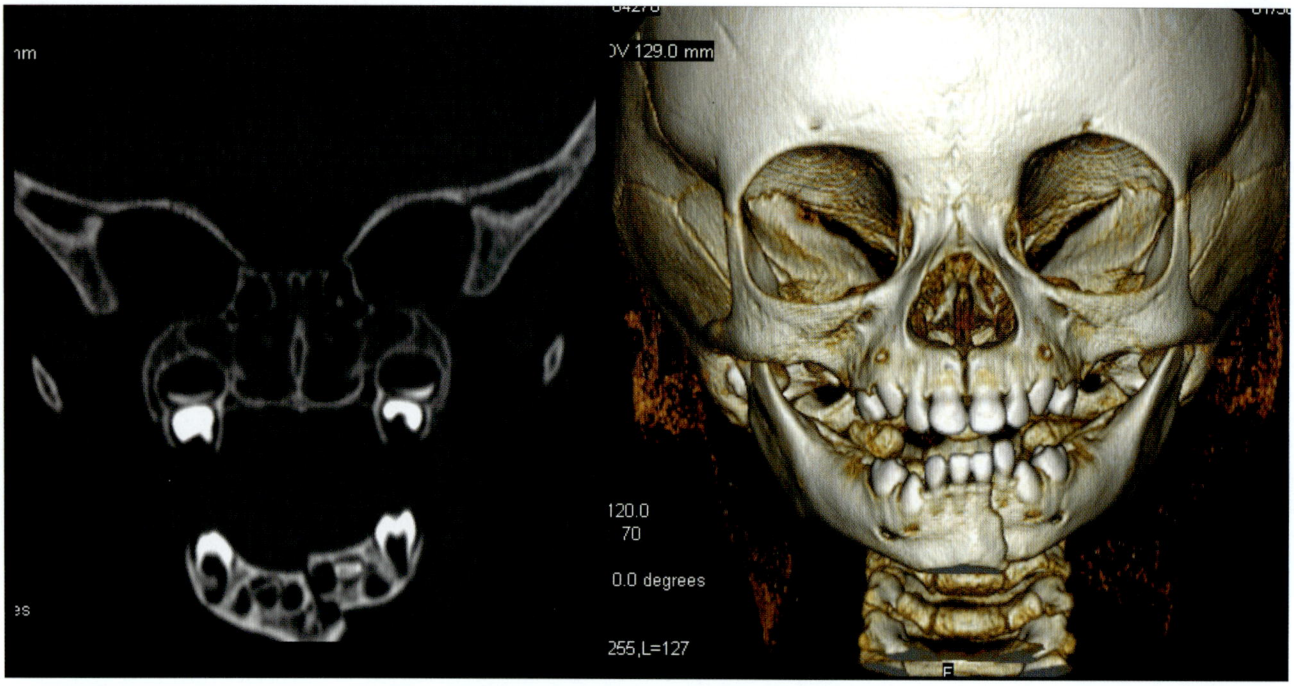

Fig 9–20. Parasymphyseal fracture. Coronal and 3-D reformations of the same fracture seen in Figure 9–19 demonstrate the superior displacement of the left hemimandible relative to the right.

on physical exam and can be proved on radiographic CT evaluation.

Before age 7, fractures of the orbital roof are more common than fractures of the floor and are often associated with frontal bone fractures (Figs 9–21 through 9–26).[2] Frontal sinus fractures also increase in frequency as pneumatization of the sinus proceeds.[2] When fractures involve the frontal sinus, evaluation of the integrity of the thin posterior wall of the sinus with CT is needed and clinically relevant due to the increased risk of central nervous system infection in association with posterior wall fractures (Fig 9–27).

Fractures of the zygomatic arch are infrequent in young children, becoming more common with maturing facial shape. Greenstick or nondisplaced fractures are most common.[1] Zygomaticomaxillary complex, maxillary, and midface fractures in general are seen in the setting of high-impact traumas such as MVA (Figs 9–28 and 9–29).[2] Before age 10, fractures of the maxilla are rare (Figs 9–30 through 9–32).[1]

In summary, when reviewing the trauma facial CT, remember to use the clues to help locate subtle fractures:

- Air where it does not belong
- Soft tissue asymmetry and swelling
- Contour abnormality of the osseous structures.

Review the images at multiple window and level settings to accentuate the osseous structures, soft tissues, and the intracranial contents.

Structures which lie in the axial plane such as the orbital floor and orbital roof are often better evaluated in the coronal and sagittal plane. Multiplanar reconstructions should be performed routinely.

Finding a facial fracture should prompt a search for associated injuries, particularly in high-velocity or high-impact trauma.

REFERENCES

1. Shapiro, AM. Injuries of the nose, facial bones, and paranasal sinuses. In: *Pediatric Otolaryngology.* 4th ed. Philadelphia, Pa: WB Saunders; 1996;1039–1052.
2. Zimmermann CE, Troulis MJ, Kaban LB. Pediatric facial fractures: recent advances in prevention, diagnosis and management. *Int J Oral Maxillofacial Surg.* 2005;34:823–833.

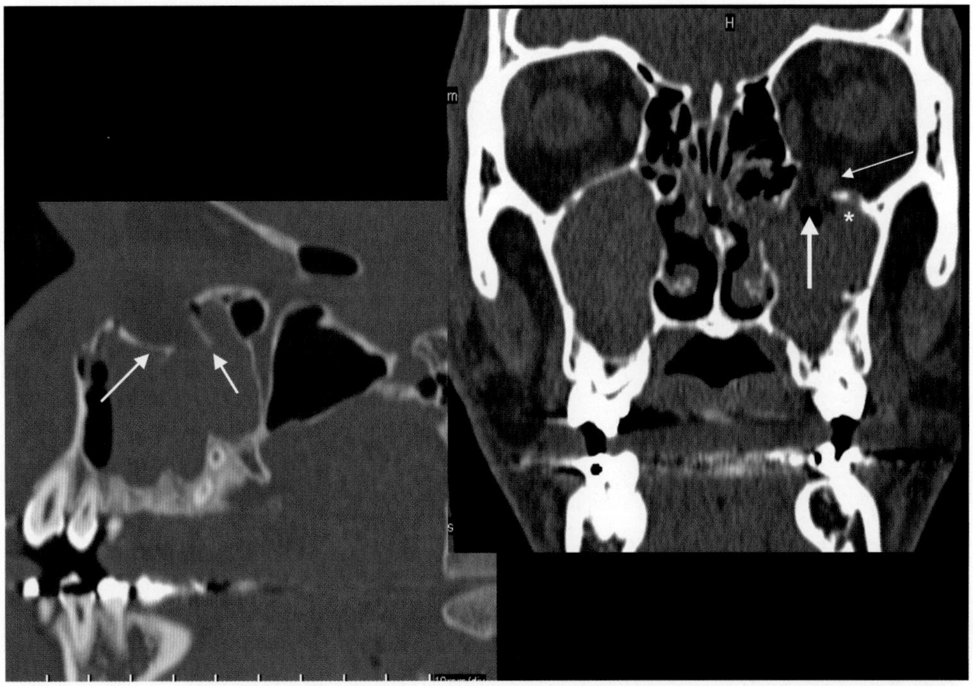

Fig 9–21. Orbital floor fracture. The image on the left is a bone algorithm sagittal reconstruction of the left orbital floor fracture and rim fracture. The inferior angulation and displacement of the anterior and posterior bone fragments into the maxillary sinus resulting in a frank defect in the orbital floor is well demonstrated. The image on the right is filmed at soft tissue window and level settings and reconstructed in the coronal plane with a soft tissue algorithm. The inferior rectus muscle (*thin arrow*) is prolapsed inferiorly into the defect as is orbital fat (*thick arrow*). The fracture line is medial to the canal for the inferior orbital nerve (*) at this level.

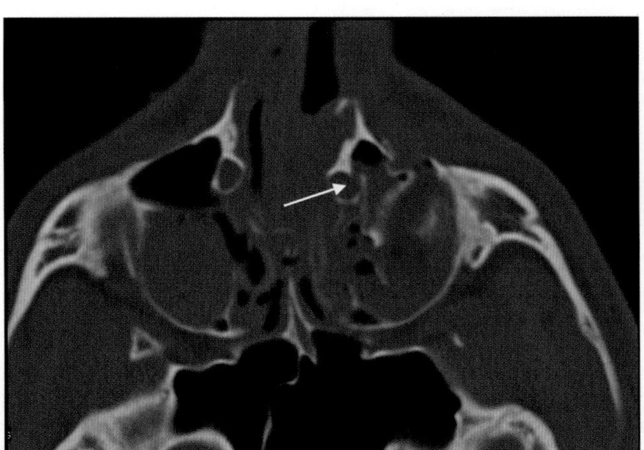

Fig 9–22. Orbital floor fracture. This is the same fracture as seen in Figure 9–21. The fracture of the floor of the orbit can be suspected by the irregular bone in the superior left maxillary sinus, but the displacement is much better demonstrated on the reconstructed images than on this axial. However, the fracture line extension to the lacrimal duct (*arrow*) is appreciated on this image.

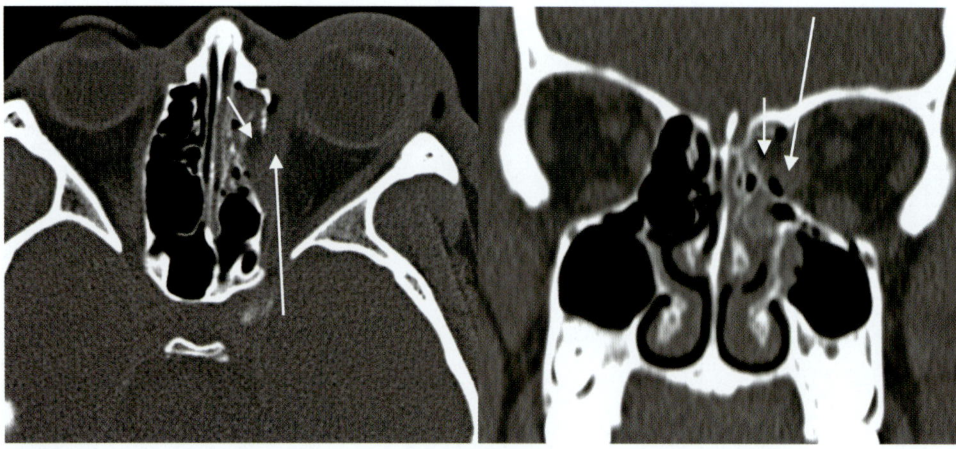

Fig 9–23. Medial orbital wall fracture. A fracture of left lamina papyracea (*short arrow*) is present. Orbital fat herniates into the defect. Also noted is thickening of the medial rectus muscle and surrounding hematoma (*long arrow*). The thin line of fat normally present external to the extraocular muscles is lost. As is best demonstrated on the coronal image, the medial rectus muscle is medially displaced into the fracture defect.

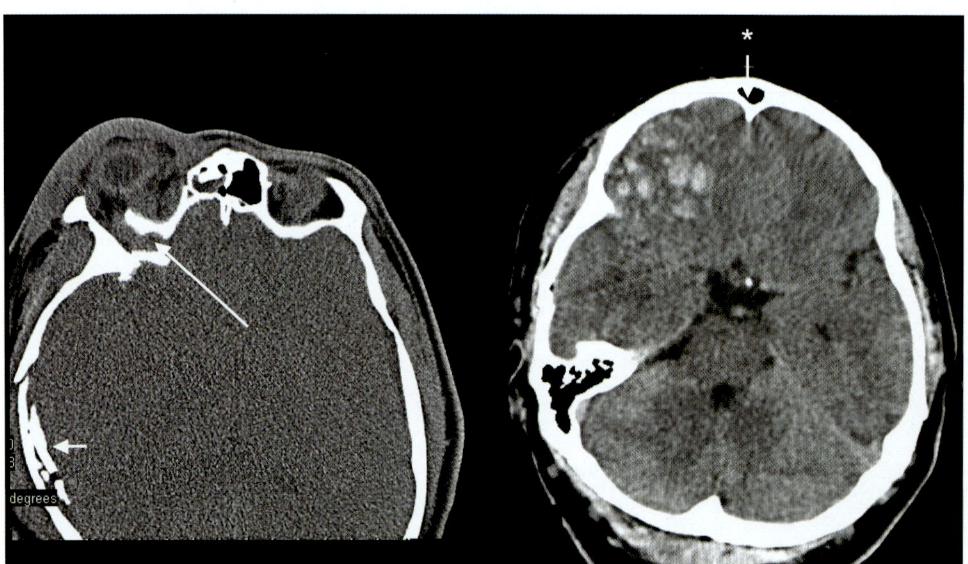

Fig 9–24. Orbital roof fracture (*long arrow*). This young patient was involved in a MVC. In the image on the left, complex right calvarial fractures are noted (*short arrow*). In the image on the right, the associated inferior right frontal lobe hemorrhagic parenchymal contusions (multifocal hyperdensities) are evident. The relatively small frontal sinus (*) is seen.

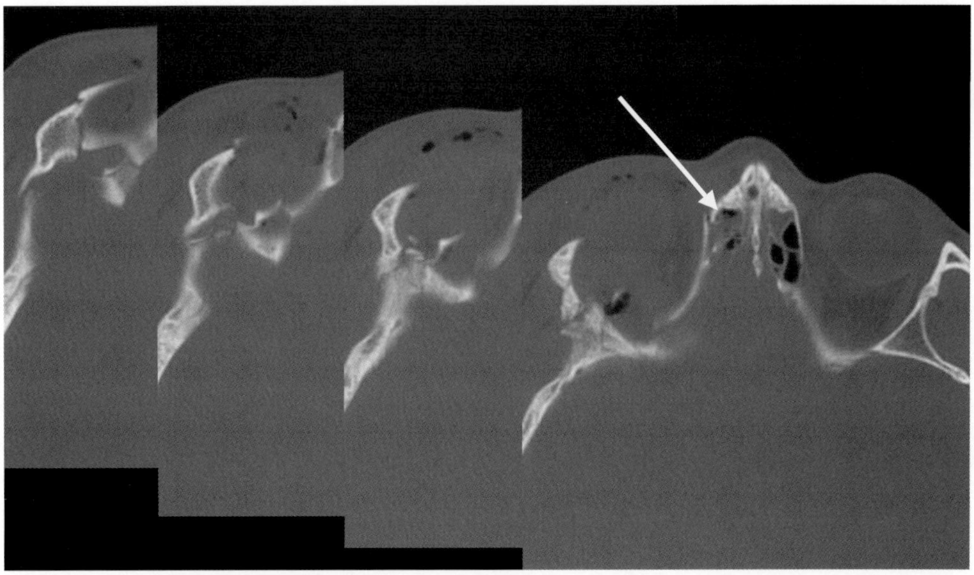

Fig 9–25. Orbital roof fracture. Four axial images from superior to inferior moving from left to right. The fracture of the orbital roof extends into the lateral orbital wall and superior orbital rim. The fracture is comminuted with free fragments and orbital emphysema. Fracture extension into the frontal recess is marked by the arrow.

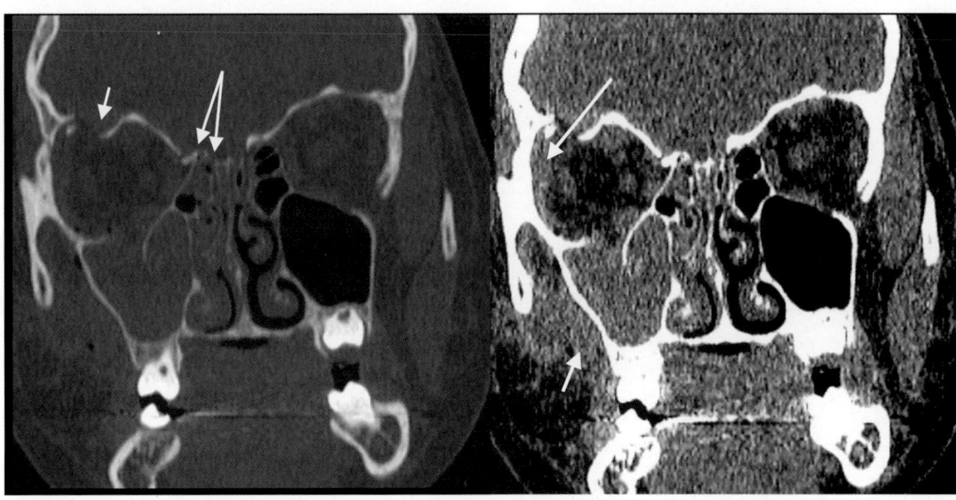

Fig 9–26. Orbital fracture. As with orbital floor fractures, these axial plane fractures are often best displayed in the coronal or sagittal plane. The two images provided are at the same location and both in bone algorithm: the one on the left displayed at bone window and level settings, the one on the right displayed at soft tissue window and level settings. The right orbital roof fracture (*short arrow, left image*) is inferiorly displaced. The right lateral lamella and cribriform plate is also fractured (*long arrows, left image*). The right maxillary sinus is opacified by blood/fluid and the orbital floor is fractured. Semilunar extraconal hematoma is seen lateral to the lateral rectus muscle (*long arrow, right image*). Hematoma is present lateral to the lateral wall of the right maxillary sinus (*short arrow, right image*).

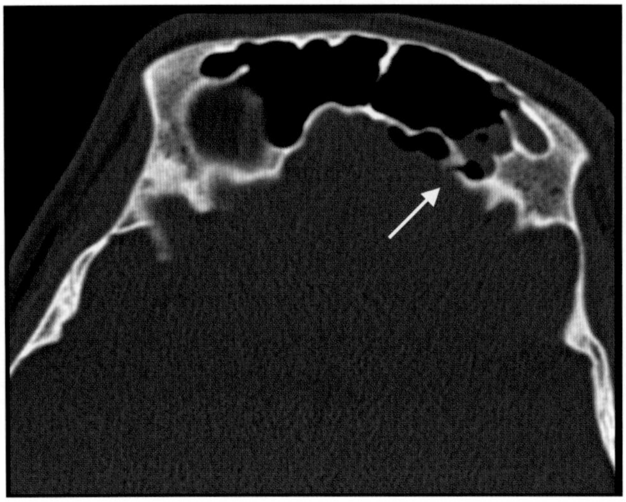

Fig 9–27. Frontal sinus fracture. This 18-year-old male involved in an MVA has well-pneumatized frontal sinuses. Not only is the discontinuity in the backwall of left lateral aspect of the frontal sinus noted, pneumocephalus is also found.

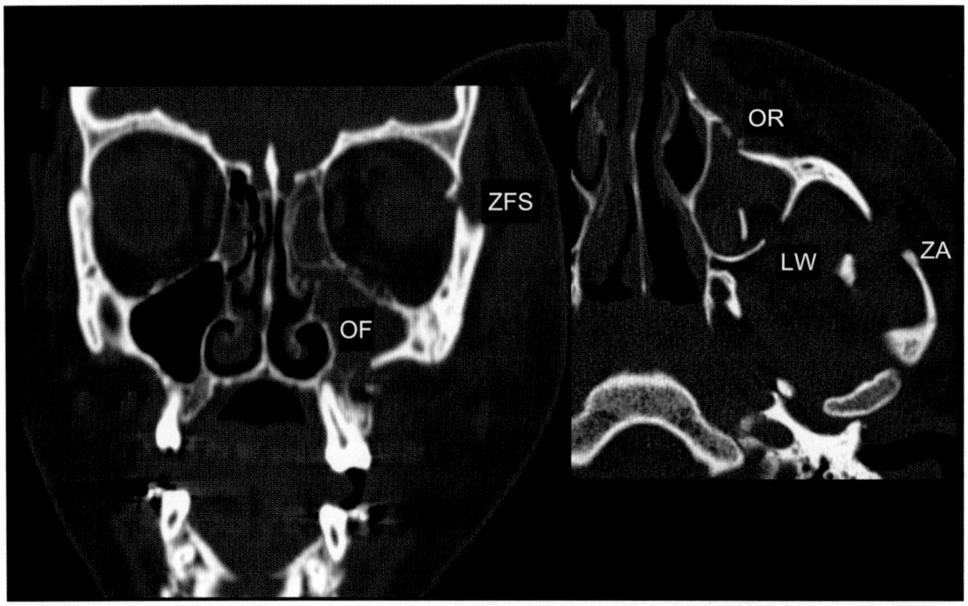

Fig 9–28. Zygomatico-maxillary complex fracture. The components of the ZMC fracture are present in this teenager involved in an MVC: fractures of the lateral wall of the maxillary sinus (LW), inferior orbital rim (OR) fracture involving the infraorbital foramen and propagating posteriorly along the orbital floor (OF), distraction and fracture of the zygomaticofrontal suture (ZFS), and fracture of the zygomatic arch (ZA).

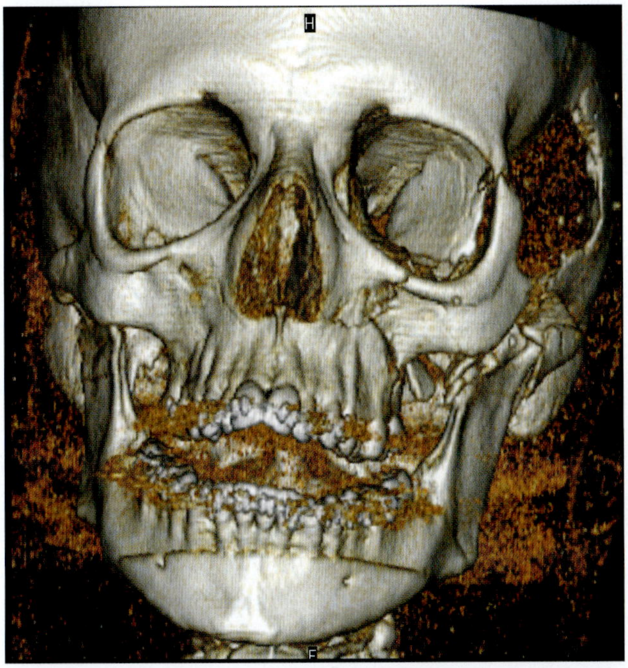

Fig 9–29. 3-D surface rendering displays the same left ZMC fracture as featured in Figure 9–28. Also appreciate the large left squamosal temporal bone defect. Incidental note is made of braces.

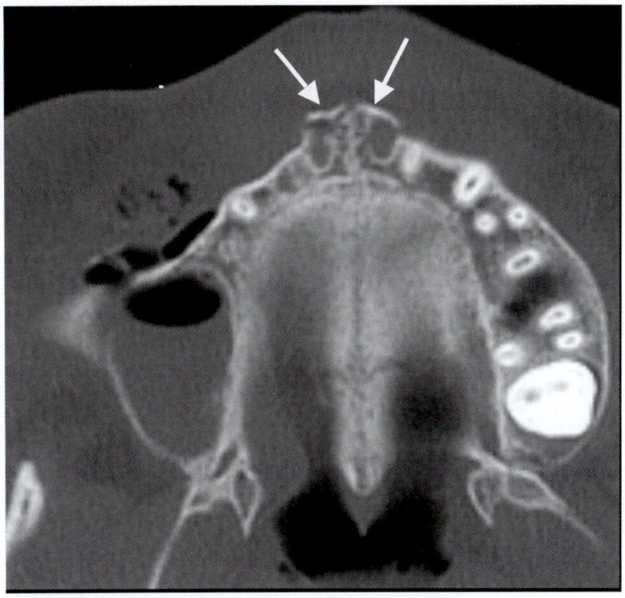

Fig 9–30. Avulsion of the central incisors of the maxilla with fracture of buccal cortex of the maxillary alveolar ridge is shown in this case. Air anterior to the anterior wall of the right maxillary sinus with an air-fluid level in the sinus raises suspicion for a concomitant maxillary sinus fracture.

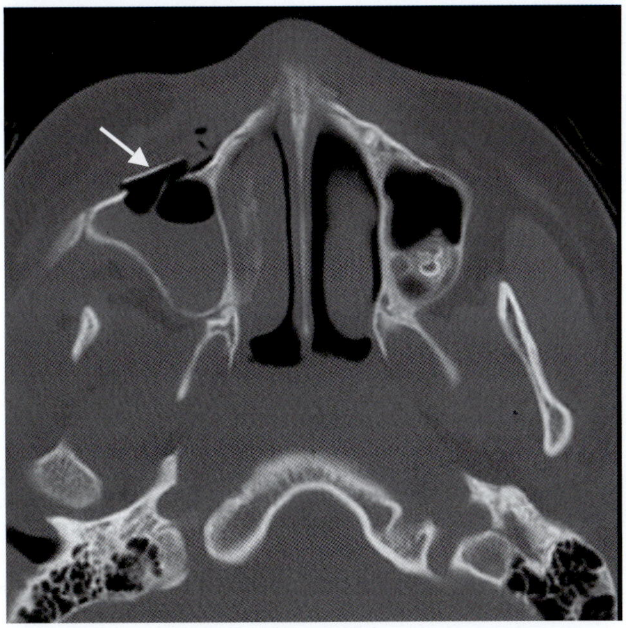

Fig 9–31. Anterior wall of right maxillary sinus fracture. This is the same patient as in Figure 9–30. A segmental fracture fragment (*arrow*) of the anterior wall of the right maxillary sinus is elevated and air is seen outside the sinus. Also note the soft tissue swelling of the right premalar location.

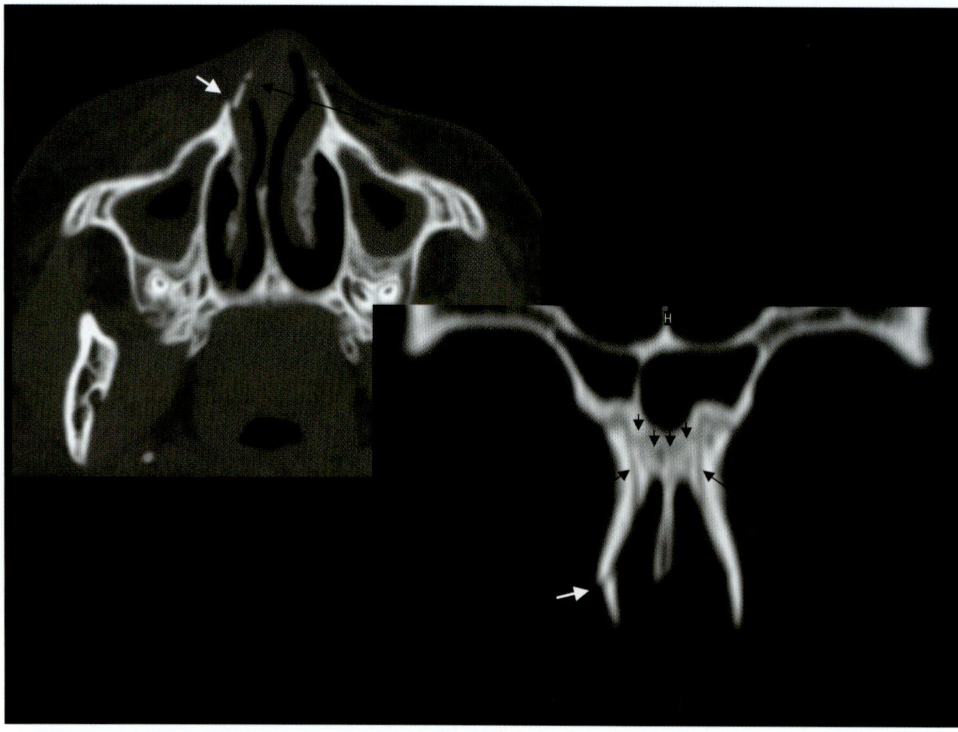

Fig 9–32. Minimally displaced right frontal process of the maxilla fracture (*short white arrow*). 15-year-old male was kicked in a fight at school. The figure on the left shows obvious right premalar soft tissue swelling and minimally displaced fracture of the right frontal process of the maxilla. The left figure is a coronal reconstruction of the same patient redemonstrating the fracture. Mucoperiosteal thickening is seen in both maxillary sinuses with an air-fluid level in the sinus on the right. Long arrows point to the nasomaxillary suture and multiple short black arrows demonstrate the nasofrontal suture on the coronal image.

Index

G

I

L

M

N

O

R

S

T

Z